OLD

Stories of Aging and Reflections on Caregiving

Rich Grimes

SUMMERLAND
PUBLISHING

ISBN: 978-0-9905886-0-3

Names of interviewees have been changed to protect personal privacy.

Printed in the United States of America.
Library of Congress #2014945150

Acknowledgements

First and foremost, I offer my sincere gratitude to the many seniors who offered time on behalf of my book, describing their lives with candor and enthusiasm. Their experiences, many of which were laced with sadness, taught me at least as much about myself as the many things I learned from them. The stories they shared and the sincere manner in which they were expressed, willingly and effortlessly, made the recording and subsequent writing a joy for me personally.

Unlike a journalist who often must search high and low seeking truth in a story, their tales resonated with a reality that moved and engaged me. Traveling miles and miles for initial and follow-up interviews proved to be advantageous as I reflected on what I should include in the text. To those individuals who helped introduce me to these amazing seniors and facilitated calendaring some of the visits, I thank you.

Family and friends played an important role in discussing, reading my drafts, and suggesting edits. My mother, Dorothy Grimes, as always, provided inspiration and words of wisdom which added levity and an earthy realism to the content. Brother David Grimes, an author himself, offered advice and editing. I much appreciate his expertise and counsel. Good friend Daniel Case provided creative ideas, many of which I incorporated into the meat of the book. In addition, he penned a very impressive foreword.

Other friends and professional colleagues whose encouragement, support, and input tightened the clarity and substance of the text include: Merle V. Stone, Dr. Bill Otto, Rene Henry, Peter Stone, Pastor Allen Hellwege, Dr. Terrence Towner, Inge Holt, Judi & Mike Nugent, Marie Ofra, Robin Karlsson, Arlene Stepputat, and Judy Fitzgerald. Also, Deanna L. Garner, Marketing & Promotions Coordinator, utilized her extensive creative talents to design a revamped website as well as other social media to publicize the book. I am grateful for her interest in and commitment to my projects.

A special, well deserved appreciation goes to Janice Blair, artist extraordinaire, who designed the cover with colors that illuminate the senses. The man's expression creates a strong curiosity to discover what is written inside.

Editing is a necessary, critical piece to reach the final product and I was very fortunate that professional editor, Michael Vizzolini, provided high quality corrections which tightened the text considerably. Thank you Michael.

Finally, credit is due to publisher Jolinda Pizzirani for her belief in my work. Her support, guidance, expertise, and accessibility kept me centered and on task as, admittedly, I struggled to write the final chapters. For that I will be forever grateful.

Foreword

Old: Having or exhibiting the wisdom of age; mature; sensible. That's one definition. Acting with or showing good sense; that's another interesting dictum. Or this one: Complete and finished in natural growth or development - worked out fully in the mind; perfected. In the vernacular, "old" just means getting up there; not a kid anymore, getting on, hanging in there, but on the way out. In Geology, old or aged means being near the base level of erosion. All right, let's not go there.

My father, 92, says, "Don't get old," when asked how he's doing. But Dad, the Bible says, "Better is the end of one's life than the beginning of it." He doesn't agree. He's tired. The Bible's words refer to the end of one's life as the true determination of worth. Even if you aren't a Biblical scholar, this statement has merit.

Within these pages, Rich Grimes introduces us to comical, cynical, educated, opinionated, but always extremely interesting elderly persons. Each will enlighten and enthrall you with candor, humor, and wisdom, revealing their strength of character, particularly overcoming personal obstacles.

Through storytelling, this diverse cast of seniors, their families and caregivers, ignite the reader to laugh out loud and cry a little; but, most important, to learn from their experiences.

As you meet Mary, Jakub, Angelica, and others you will have proof positive that the end of one's life can indeed be better than the beginning of it. Even my father, or your father, for that matter, would have you believe it. In sharing these stories, their lives are validated and celebrated. Like Rich Grimes, you just have to be willing to ask the questions.

Daniel Case, Artist – Designer – Writer
Carpinteria, California

Preface

Aging remains a perpetually popular topic, often entering conversations at will referencing a milestone birthday, a graduation, a death of a friend or family member, or someone's recent facelift. Finding humor or meaning in aging and the inevitability of death can be a bit of a stretch. My 95-year-old mother, Dorothy Marie Grimes, lives in an assisted living facility. She remains fit both mentally and physically and proved to be an inspiration in writing this book.

The definition of aging is fluid, subject to interpretation. An excellent question is *how* we are old. First, however, let's examine what is *old.* Conversing with my mother to include thoughts, quips, and wisdom to legitimize and energize the text, it occurred to me she had aged well. Her vitality and genetic composition have undoubtedly impacted her longevity. In a recent conversation, she referenced a reaction to a friendly question she often poses to a neighbor in the "institution," as she calls it. "How are you today, Phil," she inquired. His response, "I'm old." His retort is the same each time he is asked. Apparently, Phil focuses his existence on the days of his life he endures rather than those he lives. His attitude, however sad, strikes a familiar cord for many seniors.

How, then, do we define age? *Webster* offers a number of possibilities:

The part of an existence extending from the beginning to any given time.

A lifetime.

The time of life at which some qualification, power, or capacity arises or rests.

One of the stages of life.

An advanced stage of life.

The period contemporary with a person's lifetime or with his/her active life.

Generation – a long time ago.

A period of history or human progress.

An individual's development measured in terms of the years requisite for like development of an average individual.

Each definition, though commonly acceptable, somehow does not capture what I am looking for. I am not certain what a "lifetime" means due to ambiguity of the word for modern usage. In the early 19th century, the average age of a person at death was about 35. But nowadays, longevity has more than doubled. "Life times," then, depend on any number of circumstances and in an esoteric sense, age is just a word. The saying, "Time waits for no man," is true. Thus, many view time as continuing, relentless, unstoppable. Age is indeed a reality, but is aging measurable in a calendar of days, weeks, months, and years? Further, if time is an accepted continuum, we must consider that aging is logical, inevitable, and, for some, brutal. If we choose to disregard time as a measure of tracking our age, then we might have hit upon something new and exciting. That said, a new paradigm is emerging in which age is no longer an absolute. Age, after all, boils down to a number and our sense of order revolves around the recognition and celebration of special events. Mechanically, many of us accept the days of our lives as a natural progression from birth to death, but it is now clear that many variables are decelerating the aging process. These variables, one of which is improved access to health care (for some), are changing the process for good (many people are living longer), and for not-so-good (many people are living longer). I believe what is considered old and what is young overlap, with no clear-cut numerical dividing point. A litany of descriptors differentiating young and old include health, personal appearance, employment, behavior, the vehicle of choice, mental competence, mobility, and place of residence, just to name a few. But the lines between who is old and who is young have become increasingly blurred.

Views of age are often calculated by how old or young people look. Don't we all want to look younger? Not everyone, but more on that later. Exercise, a sensible diet, creams, lotions, anti-aging medications of all kinds, not to mention plastic surgery, play significant roles in physical appearance. Frankly, I can't tell with any degree of accuracy how old people are anymore. Guessing is hit or miss. I confess that from time to time, I ask a complete stranger how old he or she thinks I am – hoping, of course, for a number less than my actual age. Last year, I probed a friendly face in a restaurant and his answer made my day. "Oh, you look a lot like my brother," he said. "I think you are between 50 and 55." I responded, "Bless you, because I am 67 years old." Like many others, vanity plays a role in how old I am perceived to be by others.

According to a report compiled by 15 federal agencies, the population of older Americans is growing faster and living longer. In 2008, an estimated 39 million people in the United States were 65 or older – just over 13% of the population. Did you know that every day 10,000 Americans reach that magical, Medicare age? By 2030, when all surviving baby boomers will be over 65, the report projects there will be 72 million seniors, about 20% of the population. This statistic is staggering. The implications are far reaching in terms of Medicare, Medicaid, and Social Security costs, as well as the responsibilities of children looking after elderly parents requiring years of extended care. Individuals whose incomes during their formative years afforded a comfortable life style, including access to the best medical care, live on average 84 years, 5 years longer than those less affluent. Statistically, Americans now live longer, evidenced by the burgeoning number of us baby boomers living beyond previous norms of expected longevity.

A question arises – is living longer better? The quantity of years is one thing but the quality of those years can be something quite different. My mother's sister, Margaret recently celebrated her 101st birthday in a home where she has lived for the past 30 years. She told my mother months before that this year would be her last. My mother inquired, "Why is that?" She replied, "The money my daughter provides to keep me in this place will soon run dry, so I gotta go." We aren't sure if she was joking, but her drive to live seems to be waning. Her attitude exemplifies the inherent value of the quality of life that concerns many seniors, and begs the question – how many years are enough?

Circumstances, particularly unforeseen and unavoidable health issues, impact feelings about living and can darken the mood of even the most positive and resilient senior. Choices made when the worth of life is questioned can also impact attitude and length of life. A line in the movie, *The Shawshank Redemption*, echoes this sentiment. Oscar winning actor Morgan Freeman played a prisoner serving a life sentence, and following a friend's suicide and his own parole, he stated, "Get busy living or get busy dying." His mantra has merit.

Then, is aging a state of mind or merely a deterioration of the physical self? Both? Inactivity accelerates aging as does losing a spouse or life partner. Living alone isolates and often propels seniors into an increasingly dark state of mind, a world heretofore unknown, and not of their own choosing. Their world narrows, friends die, others move away, and for many travel is no longer an option. Lack of mobility, diminished personal association and communication with others, the monotony of a daily routine, affects mental equilibrium in a most disconcerting and disturbing way. In her book, *The Measure of My Days*, Florida Scott Maxwell states, "The old are unsure of a future and their past has grown stale." Or, she continues, "The old live by recalling the past, and are fascinated by the query of what future is possible. Their present is empty. There is nothing to be said about the old, except that they are absorbed by age." The darkness in these words is striking.

Offering a scientific prospective, in an international medical symposium some years ago on, "Death and Dying," Ven P.A. Payutto commented, "Old age and death are natural phenomena. In accordance with the law of nature all conditioned things are impermanent and liable to change, subject to causes and conditions. Everything that has a beginning must at last come to an end. The lives of all beings, after birth, must decay and die. Aging is just the decline of life and the decay of faculties; and death is the passing-away, the termination of the time of life." These thoughts resonate clearly with reasoned deduction. The actual moment of death reveals the truth of inevitability, often denied by the living.

Consistent with Payutto's assertions, Buddha said, "You need to accept that death comes in the normal course of life."

I contend that viewed separately, life and death are at odds. On the contrary, life is the *ying* and death is the *yang*, interconnected and equal. Since man was not created to live forever, the inevitability of death is a given, but the length of life is not. Unfortunately, the fear of death is often driven by questions regarding life's purpose, the uncertainty of the afterlife, and the anticipated severance from loved ones. Individuals choose to feel anxious or accepting about these concerns and one can't help but surmise worrying about them actually shortens life's years. On the contrary, in his book, *Nearing Home*: *Life*, *Faith*, *and Finishing Well*, evangelist Billy Graham writes, "I can't truthfully say that I have liked growing older, but that's just part of the realities of life as we grow older." The calming nature of Graham's words comfort and reassure.

For some age is a non-issue. James Biggs, a 104-year-old resident in a Dallas, Texas retirement community stated, "I don't think about my age. It's only a number." Many people say the same thing. I know I do. Numbers reference events: birthdays, anniversaries, days left until school ends or retirement begins, or a person's age. If aging has an evolving connotation, mere numbers are now irrelevant. On my 50th birthday (1996), my daughters wished me a happy day but said softly but with conviction, "Dad, you're old." I laughed but taken aback because I didn't consider 50 to be old at all. Going forward and validating my notion, 50 is the new 30, and 70 is the new 50, and so on. However, these calculations, most subjective of course, beg the question – why do we subtract 20 years from our actual age to determine an imaginary one? Many people 70, or even 80 or 90 years old look and act much younger than their age. Popular vocalist Tony Bennett at 88 still sings well, on key, and maintains a handsome look. Maybe aging isn't so bad after all, at least for some. But the thought of dying often pervades our thinking and can interfere with aging's natural progression. Understanding and accepting that life and death are connected is essential in assuaging our fears about exiting this time and space.

Optimists, by virtue of their "glass half-full" mentality, believe we should enjoy; in fact, relish the days we experience and not worry about tomorrow. I offer that fretting about situations and circumstances over which we have no control exacerbates the aging process. Denial of aging and our eventual death are impediments to living a life with meaning and exuberance. As Abraham Lincoln tells us, putting "life" into years can and will enhance happiness and perhaps even give us more time.

In a respectful, sincere and, at times, lighthearted manner, *Old – Stories of Aging and Reflections on Caregiving*, describes what it means to grow old as a precursor to death. However, I will not trespass on the sanctity of life warranting our unconditional reverence. Understanding that aging is seen by many as a cloud darkening their existence, others view it as a natural, sometimes welcome consequence of a life well spent. Providing a forum for seniors to look back, reflect, and share their stories will help us examine our own lives in a different and perhaps more optimistic way. A dignified life is exemplified in the concluding scene of the movie, ***The Last Samurai.*** The Samurai warriors, led by Katsumoto (Ken Watanabe) and the American Captain Nathan Algren (Tom Cruise) are defeated by the regular Japanese army, spelling the end of the Samurai forever. Algren survives but his friend is killed. The Japanese Emperor, who held Katsumoto in high regard, granted Algren an audience following the deciding battle. Injured and mourning his dead comrade, he presented Katsumoto's sword to the Emperor who asked, "Tell me how he died." Algren replied, "I will tell you how he lived."

Interviews conducted with seniors 65 years of age and older fuel the text, adding interest, depth, and meaning to questions of illness, living, aging, and dying. However, in some interviews, life is celebrated with such positivity and energy that issues of aging and death took a back seat. That said, I discovered early on that pre-determined questions compromised the story telling. Accordingly, I served as an interested listener, not a journalist, in order to facilitate an informal process of communication. The names of the seniors included in the book are confidential, and I have transcribed dialogue to personalize and illuminate my work, portions of which are fictionalized. The information contained in the stories offered by each senior surprise and inspire, and I feel privileged to have been the benefactor of their trust in sharing intimate details of their lives with me. Wise and compelling, the experiences they describe will live on for generations.

The final chapter offers an analysis of caregiving. Researching content for this book, interviewing seniors, and working as a hospice volunteer, I have been exposed to the unique world of caring for others. Caregivers in all types of situations demonstrate many admirable personal qualities – patience, kindness, flexibility, durability, adaptability, and compassion. The unselfish efforts on behalf of their loved-one or friend reach a level of unparalleled dedication, but not without frustration and uncertainty. Most learn to understand and cope well with the demands of their tasks, but adapting to the specific needs of seniors with impaired memory, particularly reacting effectively and appropriately to their language and behaviors, are daunting, to say the least. Each individual requiring care, long or short term, possesses personality traits and tendencies that fluctuate day to day. Accordingly, caregiving is not an exact science. Far from it. But those individuals who give their time, energy, and heart to others are angels in disguise.

Contents

"And in the end, it's not the years in your life that count. It's the life in your years"
-Abraham Lincoln

Chapter I – Charles (Age 92)

The interview with Charles was arranged by my church pastor. When Charles learned about my interest in interviewing senior members of the congregation for use in a book, he notified the pastor who scheduled a time for us to meet at the church ante room. Charles and I exchanged small talk prior to the interview and he was enthusiastic about the opportunity to share his life story. Tall, medium build, and balding, he appeared to be the picture of good health. Having just celebrated a happy 92nd birthday, he leaned forward to tell his story looking like a man much younger.

Responding to my first question, he thought for a moment and then stated, "Life has been good to me." I inquired, "How so?"

"Well, he said, I survived World War II, a nasty divorce, and I have worked steadily for most of my adult life. Although there have been a few ups and downs with employment, I love fixing and servicing cars so being an auto mechanic has been most enjoyable. Luckily, I have lived long enough to enjoy my four grandchildren and three great-grandchildren."

I asked, "You appear to be very healthy. Have you had any major health issues?" His answer validated his longevity. He stated, "I eat right, sleep like a baby, walk most days, still drive a car, and romance my wife. One of our favorite things to do is to share a hot fudge sundae at McDonald's, with extra hot fudge, of course. I avoid

doctors – they always give bad news." Stated emphatically with much self-assurance, I didn't ask for additional information about his health. But I wondered how a man his age could have sidestepped a disease or a major health issue.

Charles is a religious man. He stated that he has benefited from the influence of many important angels in his life – whoever they were and that the Lord protected him, shielding him from harm's way. This was validated, at least in his mind, by his assignment to an Army Air Force base at Goose Bay, Labrador in northeast Canada in 1942 following his enlistment. Nowhere near a combat zone, he served as an auto mechanic in a motor pool company. His worksite was adjacent to a refueling station for Allied bombers en route overseas where he remained for a year prior to being shipped to another assignment at Edwards Air Force base in California. While many of his fellow soldiers were sent overseas to Europe or the Pacific, he was one of only a few men who ended up back in the states as the war raged on. He thanked God for his good fortune.

He described further his involvement in the war and emphasized he had mixed emotions about serving in support of Allied troops rather than soldiering in a combat area. He realized that his skill in auto repair and maintenance was important since keeping jeeps, automobiles, trucks, and all sorts of mechanized vehicles in proper running order supported the Allies significantly in all fighting arenas of the war. However, he felt guilty at times he didn't make more of a direct contribution to the war effort. He recalled on most days while working in Canada that he watched the bomber crews take off, heading for action that was certain to be very dangerous.

Indelible on his mind, he stated, "I will never forget the sound of the engines warming up before takeoff." He then stared off and appeared a bit glassy-eyed. It was clear to me that he would forever carry the

memory of the brave young airmen who didn't return, paying the ultimate price in defense of their country. Their sacrifice helped win the war.

Although information about the locations and missions of the American crews was confidential, scuttlebutt on the base filtered around, including the nicknames of planes shot down and the fate of the crews. This saddened him very much but he realized the price for victory over the Germans and Japanese would be high in terms of injuries and lives lost. He never took his own safety for granted, believing he and his fellow soldiers were contributing in some way, albeit indirect, to ultimate victory. My research revealed slightly over 16 million men and women served in the American military during World War II, and of this number, a majority served in non-combat roles. Charles was one of the lucky ones who survived and was discharged from the Army in 1946 at the age of 25.

Since we had a natural break point, I asked his thoughts on aging and dying? Pausing briefly, he stated, "I don't think much about aging but I do think about dying." Obviously, Charles has aged well as he possesses a functional, healthy body and an alert, active mind. Aging, unlike many of his contemporaries, has not yet betrayed him. Accordingly, I postulate that aging and death are facts of life and work in harmony for a prolonged existence. Charles, well along in his evolutionary development; in fact, at the trimester of his life, is well ahead of the curve. There is no doubt Charles is making the most of his time.

Unlike many individuals who talk incessantly about aging this, aging that, friends or loved ones who can't walk or speak, or suffer from any one of many age-related maladies, he bypassed this topic and headed straight to something he feared – his own death. He said, "Death is a most interesting, scary proposition because what follows is unknown. The hereafter is a question mark

as far as I am concerned. Furthermore, there had better be a heaven but I don't know if I qualify." I thought about asking him how one qualifies, but I just let him talk.

He explained how he has prepared for his death while at the same time keeping himself organized in the present. "I have created a thorough document my attorney calls a trust. I call it my post-death decree." I asked what he meant by that. He replied, "All my finances, legal documents, divorce papers, and inheritance information on behalf of my family are contained in this decree." He indicated everything had been witnessed and signed off by all affected parties, stored in several secure locations including a safety deposit box. I nodded as he continued, "I still maintain a disciplined life with everything in its place. Ask my wife. My shirts are pressed and lined up neatly in my closet. The dresser drawers containing my underwear and socks are well stocked and organized according to color. And I bathe once a day." We both chuckled.

I couldn't resist a retort, "My mother taught me that cleanliness is next to Godliness." He agreed, smiling – "I believe that."

After a short break during which Charles and I spoke with the pastor, we sat down and continued the interview. I was developing a strong admiration for him. His candor, openness, and sense of humor juxtaposed a touching, almost child-like vulnerability. To this end, words he spoke earlier surfaced in my mind which I referenced. "You said there had better be a heaven but that you weren't sure you qualified. Can you elaborate on what you meant by this?"

He turned his head, paused, searching for words. I waited. "Rich, I am a Christian and I have led a life filled with many blessings. I have been good to others. Accepting Jesus as my Lord and Savior and following his teachings has been a cornerstone of my existence, but I remain uncertain of what will happen to my soul after I die."

In response, I asked, "What do you think happens to your soul?"

"I don't know," he whispered. A silence followed and I waited for him to continue. He then altered the topic slightly and stated, "I truly believe that an angel has watched over me."

I asked the obvious. "What makes you think so?" He then described many wonderful events of his life including his second marriage, having two special sons, and how his grandchildren and great-grandchildren have enriched his life. Contradicting slightly the earlier description of good health, he stated that a heart condition threatened his life while in his early 50s. During this experience he had sensed a comforting hand on his shoulder, guiding and inspiring him, perhaps healing him. Over 40 years ago, he felt that it was not his time to die. A key moment in the interview, I interjected, "Who or what do you think was this helping hand?"

He stated confidently, "It had to be an angel. It just had to be. I believe in them." I responded, agreeing. The initial interview concluded.

Weeks later, I re-read my notes and gave full attention to Charles' confident assessment about the benign intervention of an angel or angels in his life. I don't question his assertion but wonder if the angels he referenced were actually family members and friends whose influence on his life he has for some reason failed to acknowledge. Another theory, perhaps more reasoned, is that the Lord commissioned angels to work with his benefactors to ensure a continued existence. In this way, his purpose for living had not yet been realized; hence, he lived on. Two Biblical passages may explain the longevity Charles continues to enjoy.

The first, told to me by my dear mother, provided comfort and guidance through a personal crisis years ago, and remains a rock upon which I lean for support. Romans 8:28 states, "All things work for good for those

who love the Lord and are called according to his purpose." These words, powerful and true, relate to Charles' life as does the next passage, reinforcing his belief that an angel was protecting him. In Luke 4:10, "For it is written, he will command his angels concerning you to guard you carefully." Charles is a man of this world and of the next; kind, sincere, and loving who underestimates his good works and the benevolent intervention on his behalf provided by and through the Lord he loves so much. I am in no position to state who enters and who doesn't, but my heart and mind tell me with a great optimism he indeed *qualifies* for a place in heaven.

Nearing the end of a session lasting about an hour, I asked Charles to talk about his youth. Born in Nashville, Tennessee, in 1921, he said he didn't like school much, but he enjoyed tinkering with cars. His father was an iron worker and good with his hands. Consequently, he inherited skills that made him handy around the house. His mom relished the fact that he could fix just about anything. Seeking an opportunity that would provide increased income and sunshine to go with it, his father moved the family to Burbank, California, in the San Fernando Valley in 1938. The valley was a growing area and attracted a wave of young families looking for a better life. Both agriculture and industry provided a plethora of employment opportunities and his mother and father both landed good jobs. He helped his father at an auto repair shop after school on week days until World War II turned the world upside down. Charles was 21 years old when he enlisted in the United States Army.

He said, "I knew I had to meet Uncle Sam sometime so I didn't wait to get drafted. Boy, I was in for the shock of my life during boot camp in North Carolina. There weren't many cars awaiting repair in the swamps we had to wade through – lots of snakes and mosquitoes, though." His sense of humor was very refreshing. He went

on, "I thought I wouldn't make the grade. But as they say, "What doesn't kill you makes you stronger."

Following the war, he returned to Burbank, California, married, divorced, landed a good job at an auto repair shop (of course) a short distance from Lockheed Aircraft Company. After remarrying, the "woman of his dreams," as he phrased it, he eventually earned enough money to construct several industrial buildings in Burbank. Charles was proud of what he was able to achieve and at one time managed one of his buildings with seven employees. He stated, "We remained in Burbank through the 1980s, had two wonderful sons, and earned enough money to put money into a savings account. Many folks nowadays have never had that luxury." How right he is. Staying true to his God-given skills, he decided to branch out and perform different tasks to earn money. "I built cabinets and taught myself how to install air conditioning units in cars. But my first love remained repairing cars and got a lot of satisfaction in making them run properly. I cut back on my hours at my shop but quit working in 1991."

I inquired, "You mean you retired?" Smiling, he snapped back, "Heck no, I consider myself an unemployed auto mechanic and not retired."

Charles is a product of a unique group of individuals who saved us from the real threat of world domination by the Axis powers, keeping our way of life intact. He and the millions of Americans we often refer to as the *Greatest Generation* sacrificed much unselfishly, thousands with their lives.

He and I exchanged pleasantries and I thanked him for his time, energy, and effort sharing his story. The interview concluded with a warm handshake.

I often think about legacies: presidents, inventors, athletes, generals, teachers, doctors, philanthropists, clergy, artists, scientists, and moms and dads, just to mention a few. The more famous the individual, the

greater the legacy. However, many people we don't know, read, or hear about have quietly earned a special status. Charles is such an individual. His history of a life well lived, experiencing it with purpose, humility, great faith, and an exceptional work ethic speaks volumes about his character and shines a light on all who know and love him.

"Everyone is the age of their heart"
-Guatemalan proverb

Chapter 2 – Mary (Age 82)

A friend arranged an interview with Mary through the director of an assisted living facility on the central coast area of California. Unlike many of the residents, she volunteered admission, much to the surprise of her two grown children. Standing, she met me in the courtyard adjacent to her room, located on the first floor of a large building plastered in yellow stucco with a red tile roof. There were two fountains between lots of tables and chairs with umbrellas protecting the seated inhabitants from the sun. Slight of build with short gray hair, Mary was mobile, alert, and I would soon learn she had a warm personality. She extended her hand and greeted me with a smile.

I explained that I was gathering information from a cross section of seniors, age 65 and older, to write a book. Responding enthusiastically, she stated, "Well, we're not getting any younger. Let's get started." We shared a laugh and I knew instantly that our comfort level would facilitate a productive interview.

"Hello Mary. Thanks for meeting with me. First, please describe your personal background."

Putting on sunglasses, she stated, "Let's see, first of all, I was born in Elbow Lake, Minnesota, in 1931. Although times were tough during my childhood, at least as I can best recollect with the *Great Depression* and all, my father earned a modest income keeping our family afloat. My brother, John, three years older, kept an eye on me. My little sister, Sarah, was born in 1934, and I returned the favor, babysitting her when I was old enough

to be responsible. I loved the winters playing in the snow, and there was plenty of snow, believe me. The nights froze the socks right off us and the days weren't all that warm. But the summers were special. The weather was mild and not too hot. We three kids sold lemonade in front of our house just about every day. That was fun, but I think we drank more than we sold. Those were special times."

I then asked her to tell me about her parents.

She replied, slowing her speech slightly, "There was sadness in our house I am sorry to say. My mother, bless her, was a good person and housewife, but she was a shy, insecure woman, and when we were in school and was home alone, drank heavily. She tried to hide it but we all knew. To my father's credit, he was kind to her, very supportive and understanding, but her drinking persisted. She refused help and often went into extended moods of depression and isolated herself. She also alienated herself from friends and so they stayed away. When my brother, sister, and I reached our teenage years, my father had to take over. He did the cooking, cleaning, yard work, and helped us with our homework. My mother remained in her room days at a time. My father tried to convince her to go to counseling. She refused, and the loving and supporting words of encouragement fell on deaf ears."

Mary started to cry but continued, "As hard as my father tried, and he did try, her health deteriorated. My senior year in high school she was hospitalized and died of liver failure. She was only 45. Her death shattered our family. My father grieved a long time and never remarried."

She apologized for her tears and I shook my head and said, "That's all right. I understand." At my suggestion, we took a short break.

I second-guessed myself about asking her to describe family history. But our interaction set the stage for other personal revelations as well as establishing trust. It was apparent she wanted to talk about her mother, a

decision she made perhaps to share feelings she had bottled up for years, an emotional release. I was impressed by how well she articulated her words and guessed she was college-educated. I later learned she earned a B.A. in Communication Arts. "Mary," I asked, "As you look back in your life, what experiences or events stand out in your mind?"

She replied, "Oh, my there are so many. I recall vividly the healthy births of my two beautiful children, Michael and Meredith. Raising them was a joy and they remain rocks of support in my old age. They are wonderful."

I hesitated but asked for clarification regarding what she meant by her children's "healthy" births. She replied, "I was getting to that. In my late 20s, after earning a college degree and marrying an amazing man who, by the way, I met at a frat party, Curtis and I set up house in San Diego. We tried unsuccessfully to have children, which was very frustrating. A friend advised us to seek counseling and treatment at a fertility clinic. We did so, but the results were not favorable. Our experiences there actually increased our anxiety. My first pregnancy resulted in a miscarriage and tragically, two years later I lost twin girls due to a serious abdominal infection. My husband and I were devastated, but we recovered and decided to simply enjoy each other. Our faith made us strong. And you know what happens when you let go of bad feelings. Boom! I was pregnant again and, happily, on my 29th birthday (July 4), I had Michael and believe it or not, two years to the day, Meredith was born."

I asked how she and her husband aged. She said, "I knew that question was coming. All went well in our family. The kids were easy to parent. Michael was a good student and participated in high school sports, which kept him out of trouble. Meredith was a merit scholar and was involved in all kinds of extracurricular activities. I remember thinking that everything was too good to be

true. Curtis and I took fun vacations after the kids were grown and gone, and nearing 60, Curtis and I started planning our retirement. We were aging gracefully although I always resented the fact that despite being several years older, he looked much younger than me. His good looks and youthful spirit confirmed what I have always believed. Most men age well while women deteriorate noticeably. I hate that! But that didn't stop me from loving him. However, I sensed something was about to spoil our retirement. Don't ask me why. Turns out, I was right."

Mary's mood changed suddenly and she seemed upset. I told her she need not describe their post-retirement, but she insisted. She had a box of Kleenex anticipating an emotional outpouring, but she maintained her composure. It was obvious she wanted to talk.

"My dear husband worked hard his entire life. He was a gifted mechanical engineer for a lucrative firm in San Diego and earned an excellent income that provided our family with pretty much everything we needed. I was a stay-at-home mom. He struggled some the last two years of his employment, though. I thought he was burned out, evidenced by the travel books scattered throughout the house, but he told me otherwise. Anyway, on the anniversary of his 30th year of work, the company threw a big party for him. Well, more like a bash. My children and I attended, of course, and we shed tears of joy. Curtis looked more relieved than happy. True to form, his company awarded him a generous retirement bonus. Typical of my husband, he didn't expect anything other than receipt of his 401K in full. The frosting on the cake came at the end of the party. His boss paid him a very flattering tribute; a very nice speech, and presented him a small gift wrapped in red, white, and blue, on the company logo. It was a wrist watch."

I started to state the obvious, but Mary put her hand up and said, "No, it wasn't just any gold watch.

Much to our amazement it was a Gold Rolex. Curtis couldn't believe his eyes, nor could we. He thanked his boss profusely and said he would never take it off. He never did. I believe that occasion, next to the birth of our children, was the happiest moment of our adult lives. I wish I could say the best was yet to come, but that wasn't to be. Two years after he retired, my husband was diagnosed with Alzheimer's."

Mary's revelation hit me like a ton of bricks. She started sobbing and I tried my best to comfort her. When she recovered, I asked if she wished to postpone the interview and continue another day. She answered that we take things up after lunch, and did I mind? I told her that I didn't mind at all. She took my hand and said softly, "Come back after lunch and I will tell you more. Putting it off another day won't ease the pain."

When I returned after lunch the facility director met me in the lobby and said Mary was sleeping. "She asked me to tell you that she was sorry about her emotional outpouring, but knew you would understand. She wants very much to complete the interview and would like you to call her." I thanked her and drove home. While in my car, I thought about the deleterious impact of Alzheimer's on family and wondered how family members accepted and coped with the fact that the disease was irreversible. My knowledge of the subject was limited, but that much I knew. Once home, I researched the causes and treatments of Alzheimer's and the support options available for families and caregivers. I hoped that learning more about Alzheimer's would better prepare me for my next session with Mary.

A progressive disease that slowly destroys memory, thinking skills, and eventually even the ability to carry out the simplest tasks, approximately 5.1 million Americans have been diagnosed with Alzheimer's disease. Caring for a person with this debilitating disease can have a high physical, emotional, and financial cost. The demands of day-to-day care, changing family roles and responsibilities as well as difficult decisions regarding placement are very challenging and heart-wrenching. Spouses who raised children must confront a new parenting role caring for their afflicted loved one. This is a daunting task for sure.

I called Mary the next day and arranged a follow-up interview and hoped my research, although not exhaustive, would prove fruitful in asking questions as well as dialoguing intelligently about her late husband. I entered the courtyard and there was Mary, engaged in conversation with a female who was much too young to be a resident. Turns out, it was her daughter, Meredith, present here to support her mother. We exchanged pleasantries and I told them I was pleased that Meredith had joined us. Meredith's participation would alter my questions and the dialogue, too, providing an adult child's perspective. She proved to be a valuable resource describing her father's battle with Alzheimer's.

When we settled in our chairs, a pitcher of iced tea was brought to the table. I waited for Mary to speak and wondered if she was up to talking about her husband's bout with Alzheimer's. She did slowly and deliberately.

"Let's see," she began. Curtis' diagnosis shocked all of us, but to his credit he actually comforted me, and said everything would be fine. He made it clear he wanted to spend his remaining days with me and promised not to be a burden. His doctor was very informative and extremely kind and prescribed medications to slow down the degeneration of brain cells. He also arranged counseling for our family. My children, Curtis, and I participated although the thought of him dying haunted me night and day. My God, he was only 60 years old! That wasn't fair. But I did all I could to support and love him. I referenced every website on Alzheimer's, read carefully, took copious notes, and in the evening hours lost track of time. I went to bed in the wee hours of the morning on numerous occasions. Eventually, Curtis exhibited some of

the behaviors described in the literature: sadness, confusion, and embarrassment among them. I hoped and prayed for a miracle, but deep down I knew it wasn't going to happen. I learned to accept that his death was just a matter of time."

Meredith held her mom's hand and for a few minutes they were silent. Mary put her head down and Meredith took the lead in the conversation. She explained in very clear language her dad's diagnosis rocked their family's world. As one might expect both she and her brother transitioned mentally from denial to acceptance. Strangely, they both were relieved when they reached the conclusion that their father was going to die. She said that they understood that supporting their mother was the most important thing they could do.

"Michael and I had many talks in the beginning about how we could help without being intrusive and we committed to learning as much about Alzheimer's as we could and focus on the support process."

I asked what that process entailed. "Once we accepted the reality of our dad's condition, we focused on helping our mom cope, remaining strong and offering our time. But we weren't sure how we could help because mom needed much more than moral support. Dad would need care and we refused to permit mom to shoulder that responsibility by herself. It would overwhelm her. A close friend whose mom contracted Alzheimer's told me that hospice care should be considered. I gave her idea serious thought and contacted the local hospice provider and spoke with the director. She was very knowledgeable and supportive. She requested our doctor contact the lead hospice physician to discuss treatment options and placement. He did so immediately."

Speaking rapidly with emotion, she elaborated. "I met with the medical team at the hospice unit later that week and, fortunately, all the appropriate medical personnel were in attendance, including both doctors. The

team recommended placement in the program and thought home care best. The individuals who monitored my dad were exceptional. They were compassionate, efficient, and highly skilled professionals. The hospice volunteer was especially nice, interacting with my dad in such a positive way and made him laugh. After a few weeks of professional, medical support and supervision, we were convinced we had done the right thing placing dad under the hospice umbrella." Meredith's voice now broke and it was her mom's turn to comfort her.

I asked the ladies if they wanted to break or stop for the day. With her head up grasping a Kleenex wiping her eyes, Meredith had more she wanted to say. "At the urging of our dad's nurse case manager, we contacted a local Alzheimer's support group and attended bimonthly meetings. We learned so much and felt reassured that we weren't the only family facing a similar circumstance. The support leader welcomed us warmly at the first meeting and distributed a packet of information listing available support resources. Those in attendance sharing feelings about their loved ones touched our hearts. Not unlike Alcoholics Anonymous meeting, there was an outpouring of emotion in the room. People spoke out, often interrupted by their own tears. Sharing made my brother and I feel better. We weren't alone."

Meredith paused and I asked Mary if she attended these meetings. She said no. "Curtis wasn't displaying visible symptoms of memory loss in the beginning, but I just didn't want to leave him alone." Mary and Meredith shared a smile.

This conversation was very powerful and draining. We had reached a point calling for a break and I wondered if asking Mary to tell more of her story was a good idea. Perhaps it would be best to defer discussion of Curtis' deterioration and focus on Mary's life after his death. Meredith gave me her cell phone number and I told her I would call to seek her advice on where to go from

here. The story certainly had more, but telling it was taking its toll on her mother.

Our phone conversation lasted more than an hour. Via speaker phone. Meredith and Michael took turns and each described in their own way how difficult it was to watch their father succumb to a condition over which no one had control.

Michael stated, "The symptoms, mild at first, accelerated rapidly and in less than a year, even with our assistance, mom couldn't adequately care for him. He had trouble bathing and was disoriented most of the time. He repeated questions after they were answered and shook his head like we were treating him as a child. The fact is that he regressed to a nearly infantile state and had to be monitored 24-7. Mom was worn thin and my sister and me spent many nights after work taking care of him. We had to force her to go out and her best therapy was having dinner mid-week with her friend, Betsy."

Meredith spoke next. "We soon realized our dad needed hospice at a facility before mom completely lost her mind. The expense was reasonable under Medicare. The hospice team concurred, and we placed him in a memory loss unit close to home where he received exceptional care. He was only 62, but life was being squeezed out of him. His system soon shut down and after only a few weeks, he died of liver and lung failure. As sad as we felt, we knew this was a blessing. His suffering ended and mom could find peace."

The phone conversation was cathartic. Meredith and Michael were incredibly supportive of their mother and did all that was humanly possible to help her endure the most difficult days of her life – evidencing their courage, stamina, and resolve. They were and are models of unconditional love. Meredith asked if I needed more information for my book. I answered in the affirmative, but only if she was willing. She said she would talk to her mother and get back to me. Several days passed and

Meredith called to tell me her mom wanted to continue our sessions.

Our final interview took place back at the courtyard near Mary's residence. She seemed more relaxed and energized, and I had her full attention. I asked about events in her life since Curtis' death. She stated, "I grieved for a long time, but family and friends coached me through it. But accepting his passing was very difficult. As you know we had plans to travel and enjoy our retirement. Living alone wasn't what I envisioned, but I have managed over the years to use my time constructively, working part time, participating in a reading club, playing tennis, and volunteering at a homeless shelter. Honestly, I probably would not have done these things if Curtis were alive. My friends, several of whom are widowed like me, have been extremely supportive."

I asked, "Did you remain in your house or move?" She answered, "Funny you should ask. I had mixed emotions about remaining in our home. I wanted somehow to keep Curtis' memory alive and keeping the house seemed the right thing to do. I have to say though that it took over a year before I could muster the courage to clean out his closet. I hadn't even opened it. Meredith, bless her, helped me but we both cried the entire time. Michael moved his dad's dresser and personal items to the garage. Once completed and after donating his clothes to Goodwill, I felt a sense of closure. Relieved, it was time to get on with my life."

Mary anticipated my next question. "If you were going to ask if I re-married, the answer is no, I didn't." She explained that she had no desire to date.....giggling. "Turning back the clock, when I was nearing 70, I just didn't want to make the time and effort to meet someone new. I know some widows hate living alone and seek a companion, but I knew no one, absolutely no one, could come close to replacing my Curtis. Besides, I grew to like

my independence. Planning each day and doing what I want, when I wanted, was a routine I enjoyed. I guess that is selfish in some ways, but I didn't want to complicate my life again. At my age, and, by the way, I will be 83 next week; one has to think about illness, either my own, or a partner. I simply have no desire to caregive for anyone again. The emotional and physical toll is too high."

"Mary," I stated, "It has been a pleasure and privilege to meet you and I am very grateful you shared your life with me. I know it wasn't easy. I also owe a debt of gratitude to your wonderful children. They are special people. Just one question remains……how do you feel about your own death?"

Mary paused, and said confidently, "Death is a reality we all must accept," she said. "We enter this world alone and leave the same way. Each of us is presented an opportunity to do good works. I am not afraid of dying. In fact, I am at peace with it. My husband's death made me realize each day is a gift and a blessing to be treasured. But all things come to an end. There is something I know for sure. I will reunite with Curtis in the next life. He is waiting for me."

The interview concluded. I expressed my deep appreciation for her time and effort, stood and gave her a hug. Mary and her children exemplify all that is good in caring for a loved one. Mary is a dear person; a good woman, wonderful mother, and loyal wife. I learned much from our experience together. Suffering great pain, a strong resilience helped her rebound from an unimaginable loss.

"He is so old his blood type was discontinued."
-Bill Dana

Chapter 3 – Jakub (Age 101) & Elise (Age 96)

While having coffee with my friend, Anne, at Starbucks, the conversation shifted from family, education, and our previous marriages, to this book. I informed her that much of the content would be derived from interviews with seniors sharing their life stories. I was delighted to learn that Anne worked part-time coordinating food services at a nearby assisted living facility. She indicated that many of the senior residents were interesting people; a diverse group she thought might like to share their stories. I welcomed this opportunity and within a week, she arranged for me to speak with a man born in 1912, the same year Woodrow Wilson was elected president of the United States.

Jakub phoned about a week later and said he and his wife wanted to be interviewed. While talking to him, I heard a voice in the background, "Speak up Jakub, he can't hear you." I asked him who that was, and he said, "That's the boss." So with a bit of humor and early insight into who ran the show, my journey began to trace the life experiences of what proved to be a most fascinating pair.

I drove to the residence facility a few days later and was impressed with the appearance of the buildings and grounds. Modern, colorful structures, there were numerous units occupying a huge area separated by beautifully landscaped gardens with paved walkways, tables and chairs appropriately located, and red

umbrellas. This was an upscale senior residence. Jakub met me in the lobby, smiled, and said he was glad I had come. Steadied by a cane, he appeared frail, but offered a firm handshake. He was tall, thin, with a goodly amount of gray hair.

He led me down a hallway past a spacious lobby entrance with cozy lounges on either side, to his apartment, turned, and said something curious. "The longer we live, the more pressure there will be on our children. The way it is now there won't be a balance." Longevity, both pros and cons, as well as its impact on family generations, surfaced in our conversations. We walked into his unit, and I was greeted by Jakub's wife, seated in a wheelchair. Elise had short, gray hair, sparkling brown eyes, and smiled as I introduced myself. She motioned for me to sit in a big, comfortable chair near the glass slider, and at the same time Jakub took a seat in what appeared to be his special chair. It was apparent they were eager to talk.

I directed my initial question to Jakub, but asked Elise to interject comments at any time. She did, correcting some of Jakub's statements. On one interchange following a remark by her husband, she looked at me and said, "Well, that's not quite right." She gladly served as the interview fact checker. Too funny!

Jakub stated he was born April 14, 1912 in Minnesota, 11 days before the sinking of the Titanic. Although he would later complain about his age, partial loss of sight and hearing, he was proud that his birth nearly coincided with an event of such magnitude. Both he and Elise attended the University of Minnesota where they met at a fraternity party. Elise smiled at his recollection, but shook her head slightly, stating, "I am not sure where we met. It was so long ago, but it was love at first sight." They glanced at each other and smiled. This was the first evidence of the bond between the two. Marrying in 1941, a month prior to the Japanese attack on Pearl Harbor, they

will celebrate their 72nd wedding anniversary this fall. Yes, that long. Incredible! I asked why the marriage had defied time. Jabuk said they were compatible and liked each other despite differences in their personalities. Perhaps opposites do attract.

Elise stated she is confined to a wheel chair as a result of a fall a few months previous, resulting in a broken hip. Turns out her immobility was the reason the couple moved from their Santa Barbara home.

She stated, "I was born in North Dakota in 1916, attended high school there and decided to pursue a college degree. Minnesota was a very affordable state university and offered a degree in law. At first, I wanted to pursue a career in tax law, but having a family changed all that." Jakub then spoke out on behalf of his wife, stating that she earned her law degree in 1940, the only female who passed the Minnesota State Bar Exam that year.

Elise then described the status of women in her day, stating that females, even those with college degrees, were discouraged, discriminated against, really, from applying for or holding professional positions.

"When women applied for employment, jobs were plentiful. If they checked the box on the application they could type, they were hired. Companies were populated by men who served in executive or management positions while women were relegated to semi-skilled, hourly jobs such as typists, clerks, and secretaries. It was a man's world at that time and I think it still is." Jakub, smiling, added emphatically, "My wife is a militant feminist." We all laughed. I then asked, "Militant is a strong word now isn't it?"

He replied, "Well, she is a very strong woman." I had no doubt he was right and now understood fully why he referred to her as the boss.

I asked Jakub if he served in the military during World War II. He stated he was exempt due to his technical educational background and knowledge of

fighter aircraft design and operations. He earned two degrees from the University of Minnesota, a B.S. in Engineering and an M.S. in Physics. He explained that after his marriage to Elise, they settled in Indianapolis, Indiana, where he was recruited and soon employed by the Allison Division of General Motors. He stopped momentarily.

My guess is he didn't want to boast about his engineering skills. However, I kept the topic alive and asked him what tasks he performed at G.M. Somewhat reluctantly, he stated that he helped design the Allison V-1710 aircraft engine used by various American fighter planes including Lockheed's P-38. Post-interview research confirmed that the P-38 served as both an attack and escort fighter in European and Pacific theatres during the war. Very fast, extremely maneuverable, and versatile, the plane proved to be a nemesis of the German Luftwaffe. The V-1710 aircraft engine that Jakub helped design and build was the only indigenous American - developed V-12 liquid-cooled engine to see service in the war.

I posed a final question about the war. "Which enemy did you fear the most?" He thought for a moment and stated, "I was most concerned about the Germans due to their advanced technology. Their rocket scientists were brilliant. The V-1 and V-2 were serious threats to the allies and world security."

Jakub spent his entire professional career as an engineer, working for G.M. in three locations – Indiana, Michigan, and a plant in Goleta, California. His skill, dedication, and work ethic underscore the contributions made by thousands of non-military personnel that helped win the war.

Seguing to a new topic, I asked Jakub to describe any fond memories he recalled. He then leaned back, thought for a moment, and said, "Fate has smiled on us." Looking at his wife, he continued, "We have remained in good health and are blessed with two grown sons, one

granddaughter, and three great grandchildren." He then moved out of his chair and pointed to pictures on two walls in their apartment of his family and named each person with a little help from Elise. Jakub then addressed a question I wanted to explore and without prompting, he stated, "Aging wears on you," and then, laughing at a line he recalled from Robert Browning, who wrote, "The best is yet to come." He looked at me and said he disagreed with Browning and stated that the best was behind him. Actually, Browning's exact words were "Grow old with me, the best is yet to come." It is interesting to note that on my second interview, Elise said Jakub was a pessimist by nature, but I would learn during the course of our experience together that he was more of a realist. I found him to be honest, forthcoming, and, understandably concerned about his deteriorating hearing and vision. He said with a frown, "Everything is wearing out."

After a brief break, inspired by the handsome family in the pictures Jakub referenced, I asked him to provide more details. Jakub's parents were born in Czechoslovakia and immigrated to America prior to the outbreak of World War I. His father, Josef, was trained in the Austrian Army and it was not known if he would have been forced to serve in the war because he was 38 years old in 1914. His parents married in America and settled in Queens, New York, moving several years later to Minneapolis, Minnesota. Jakub didn't remember how they met, but stated that his mother, Annushka, was 19 years younger than his father. He stated many marriages of Eastern Europeans united couples with the man much older. When asked what was important in his father's life, he said, "His Czech background." Then he shared a story about his father, apparently quite vivid in his memory. "When I was in 1st grade, there was an Influenza epidemic in the country and my father kept me out of school for two weeks, just to be safe. At home, he read stories to me. I think my favorite was *Molly and Polly*. He read to me in

his native Czech language with a pronounced accent. I enjoyed my time with him. When I returned to school my classmates made fun of my new accent and I made a special effort to get rid of it in a hurry, "Jakub explained. Despite a few health issues, it is quite apparent Jakub has been blessed with a memory that has not deteriorated to the degree of others his age or even younger. Family genetic make-up continues to serve him well. His recall is incredible as is his wife's.

I turned to Elise and asked her to talk about their children. She stated they had two sons who were more alike than different. "Although I had professional career ambitions," she explained. "I loved being a stay-at-home mom. I helped William (now 68) and Greg (now 62) with schoolwork, attended their school functions, and provided the guidance and nurturing I believe shaped their personalities. They turned out to be kind, respectful, and loving, and still are." Proudly, she told me both boys graduated college and work in professional capacities.

She stated that Jakub did his part, too, but he worked long hours and his job was demanding due to the urgency of the tasks he performed. Willingly, she was the glue that kept the household together and they parented with patience and understanding. She went on to say, "We were consistent and worked as a team because, as you know, raising kids is very challenging. As the boys reached their teenage years, they learned that they couldn't play one of us against the other. They didn't always like the rules we enforced but ultimately, when they became young men, they thanked us for being good parents."

I asked for more information about their sons, and she indicated that both benefited from the quality education they received from prestigious universities. William earned his B.A. Degree from Stanford University and his law degree from U.C. Berkeley and has been a successful criminal attorney for many years. William has one daughter, Jennifer, who recently received her M.B.A.

from Harvard University. She and her husband have three young children and live in Boston. William and his wife live in Pacific Palisades. Younger son, Greg, is a U.C. Berkeley graduate, single, and owns a small accounting business in Orange County. He resides in Redondo Beach. I said to Elise, "You must be proud of your sons and what they have accomplished. "Yes, very much so," she replied. I was impressed with the educational achievements of the entire family, opening doors resulting in professional success.

The initial interview with Jakub and Elise was informative and stimulating. The subsequent conversation was raw, revealing ideas of high interest. Little did I know my first question, directed at Jakub, would open a Pandora's Box.

"What happens after death," I inquired. Jakub responded immediately. "Nothing, absolutely nothing. The lights go out. End of story," he commanded in a strong voice. His expression was animated and definitive, contrasted with previous statements he made which were very gentle. As I penned his remarks, without prompting, he voiced his views on specific aspects of the Bible.

"Vanity is vanity," he stated, and I waited for him to explain what he meant. He referenced Ecclesiastes and stated life is temporary. My research revealed that the Hebrew term *hebel*, translated vanity or vain, refers concretely to a "mist," "vapor," or "mere breath," and metaphorically something that is fleeting or elusive. He then stated that he grew up in the Catholic Church but didn't buy into its beliefs nor, in his words, the "apocryphal stories" described in the Bible. He said Noah's Ark was a bunch of bologna. Conversely, he commented, "Some parts of the Bible are good and wise, especially Psalms." He expressed a great appreciation for the Bible as literature but not for its religious tenets. I asked him to talk further about religion. He did so and punctuated his words with passion.

"Religion has been the cause of war and strife for centuries and the root of many of the problems in the world today. Look at all the issues with terrorism; killing in the name of religion. This makes no sense, but organized religion is dying out. This is a good thing and down the road, not in my life time of course, the peoples of the world will come together in peace and be kind to one another. Human dignity will be restored." He then leaned back in his chair and was silent.

I turned to Elise and asked her to comment about life and death. In a calm tone, she said, "I still enjoy life and take the time to look outside our apartment and enjoy the flowers and the beautiful mountains in the distance. Life is a game." I asked, "How so?" She replied, "A friend told me once that life has 4 innings: our childhood, youth, middle age, and old age and there was a purpose in each stage. I believe that and don't regret being in the last inning – not at all. Death comes to everyone and taking one day at a time works best for me. With few health issues, I worry more about our accountant and how he is managing our estate than when I will die." She paused and then said, "As you can see, my husband is a non-believer. Jakub remained silent and didn't acknowledge her comment.

"My parents emigrated from their native Russia in 1913, and settled in a small town in North Dakota. I was confirmed in the Lutheran Church but rejected its practices. I knew Jakub didn't believe in God when I married him. I evolved into an agnostic, but accept that others, including my children and granddaughter, know and love God. I am not at that place, whether good or bad."

Jakub and Elise exemplify longevity in age and marriage. Loving, intelligent, highly educated, affluent, parents, grandparents, and great grandparents, the length of their lives could be described as a modern miracle. They are still in possession of their mental faculties and

their general health is quite good. Don't you find it incredulous they have lived 197 years between them? Kudos to this amazing couple!

"A man is not old until regrets take the place of dreams"
-John Barrymore

Chapter 4 – Lester (Age 75)

Although I recently moved to Ventura, California, last year I lived in Carpinteria, a beautiful beach city located in California's central coast, south of Santa Barbara. At that time little did I know a neighbor residing just a block away would provide both a tragic and hopeful story I would include in my book. I was most fortunate that our paths crossed the same day we were both scheduled for a medical procedure.

***Help*, a local transportation service, sent a vehicle to pick us up as we both had an appointment at a Santa Barbara clinic. Lester no longer drives and I was instructed by my doctor that I could not drive to or from the clinic due to the anesthesia used in my procedure. We got into the sedan simultaneously and occupied the back seat. After a few minutes, the driver informed us that Lester and I would be going to the same location. I asked the stranger seated next to me what he was having done. His reply offered a clue into his apparent abrasive personality.**

"That is my business," he blurted. The driver looked into his rear view mirror to watch what proved to be a very interesting, brief dialogue. I responded, "Fair enough, but would you like to know why I am going to the clinic?" Lester paused, looked me straight in the eye, and with a sarcastic tone this time, said, "Only if you wish to tell me." I explained that I was seeing a G.I. specialist who was to perform an endoscopy to determine why I was

experiencing internal bleeding. Before Lester could respond, the driver stated, "I had a similar condition a few years ago. Turns out, it was a bleeding ulcer, but the doctor eliminated it with some strong medication." Lester managed to nod his head, offering no comment.

The rest of the 15 minute trip to the clinic was void of any conversation. I surmised that Lester was repressing an emotional issue of some kind, or merely didn't want to participate in small talk with someone he didn't know. But I thought he might be an excellent person to interview. When we arrived at the clinic, the driver opened the back doors and Lester and I got out. We walked side by side in silence to the reception area. I thought that now was the moment to ask him. "Lester, I wish you well with your procedure." I told him I was writing a book on aging and dying, and asked if he would be willing to be interviewed. He stopped and much to my surprise, he said, "Why not? Maybe you write better than you talk." I suppressed a laugh and asked if I could visit him in the next couple of days. He said, "Well, you know where I live. Suit yourself." We checked in at the counter and went our separate ways. I noticed he had a slight limp, favoring his right leg. I was pleased this grumpy old man seemed willing to play along with my request. By the way, our procedures went well.

In a few days at mid-morning, I walked to Lester's apartment and knocked on the door. I was a bit nervous, hoping he would recall agreeing to see me, and wondered if his behavior would be mellow enough to make good use of my time.

He opened the door and said sternly, "I knew it was you. Come in." He invited me to sit in a comfortable, padded rocking chair. I looked about and viewed a neat, clean, and shipshape apartment, not exactly what I expected. I paused, thinking he would initiate a conversation. However, seated in the living room on a blue couch, he just stared at me. After a few moments, he said,

"Well, what do you want to know?" Sensing my hesitation, he added, "Mr. Grimes, I don't have all day." I wanted to ask him what he did all day, but I didn't think that would go over so well considering his volatile behavior during our trip to the clinic. I explained the content and purpose of my book, emphasizing stories senior share. He nodded and said, "Do you want the real version or should I make stuff up?" I replied, "Please, Lester, make it real." Without hesitating, he stated, "I shall, then."

I asked him where he grew up. "Is that the best you can come up with?" he shot back. At this moment I decided the interview would not continue unless he cooperated and eliminated his negativity. I said, "Lester, I have not said or done anything to offend you, and if you don't want to be interviewed, that is fine with me. My book will be written with or without you." Putting down my pen, I prepared to leave. Lester cracked a smile, sighed, and said in a normal tone, "O.K. Mr. Grimes, I will try to be nice.

"Excellent, then let's get started," I said. "Do you want me to repeat my first question?"

"No, that won't be necessary. I will describe my upbringing," he replied in a relativity soft tone of voice.

Lester stated he was born in Bristol, Connecticut, in 1938. He was raised by a single mother. He never knew his father and his mother didn't talk about him, as if he never existed. Having two siblings, one younger sister and an older brother made things hectic around their small house. The family of four had to make due with two bedrooms and one bathroom so privacy was minimal.

"My mom worked as a clerk at the county courthouse – a decent job, but paying the rent, utilities, feeding and clothing us was difficult, yet she never complained. She had to be frugal and expected us to help out with chores. We did so willingly. After working all day, she cooked great meals. At dinner we sat around a small oak dining room table and had some lively conversations. My mom, bless her, was a good woman."

Lester lowered his head and asked if we could discuss another topic. I said yes and it was obvious that he felt uncomfortable talking about his childhood, particularly his mother, which was an issue that would surface in our subsequent interview. I thought perhaps Lester's rough exterior had its roots in his father abandoning the family.

Providing a change as requested, I asked Lester to describe his high school days in Bristol and the events that followed his graduation. He indicated that he was, in his words, "Pretty much a loner, earned average grades, and didn't participate in athletic or extra-curricular activities." When asked if he was interested in any of the subjects he took in school, he said he enjoyed the metal and woodshop classes because the projects required tapped his natural ability to work with his hands. However, he didn't like the core classes and struggled, particularly in English. "I think I only got one grade higher than a "C" in English and math, but all I wanted was a diploma. Heck, our grades weren't written on it so it didn't matter." After graduation, Lester was hired as a mailroom attendant at a local newspaper and moved up the ladder to assistant circulation manager in a short time. He stated he followed directions to the letter, never missed a day of work, and his bosses liked his work ethic. As long as he contributed to room and board, his mother let him live at home, but he moved out after his 19th birthday into a room across the street from the newspaper. He couldn't afford to buy an automobile, so this was an ideal arrangement. When Lester met a girl his same age at a church social, his life turned upside down.

"Marjorie was the most beautiful girl I had ever seen and it was love at first sight," he reminisced. "She worked part-time and attended the local college in the hopes of becoming an accountant. She had a playful,

outgoing personality, and was very intelligent. I couldn't resist her. Her parents liked me and seemed impressed that I had a regular job at the newspaper. They invited me over every Sunday for dinner and as I recall, like my mother, Marjorie's mom was an excellent cook. Her pot roast and lemon meringue pie were to die for," he said with a forced smile on his face.

After just six months of dating, Lester asked for Marjorie's hand in marriage, and she said yes. "Asking for a *woman's hand* was the proper etiquette in those days, you know. Hell, now most couples live together and never marry, and if they do, the man doesn't ask the women's parents' permission. The world has gone mad," he barked out in a cynical tone. Much to his amazement, despite their youth, Marjorie's parents consented to the marriage with no reservations. Lester's mother and siblings, John and Sarah, and his cousins were thrilled. His family adored Marjorie. The couple had a small ceremony, a modest reception, and honeymooned in Cape Cod just for the weekend since both had to get back to work on Monday. All went well until a tragedy struck which haunted Lester the rest of his life.

Lester and his new wife rented a furnished apartment a few miles outside of town. "Playing house," as Lester described it, was fun and they looked forward to a long life together. They settled into a routine that suited their work and school schedules. "I even learned to cook," Lester said, "Out of necessity since Marjorie attended business classes two nights of the week. I refused to use a cook book, at least at first, and I burned several dinners before I realized that preparing a meal was much different and in some ways more challenging than changing the oil in my car." Lester backtracked at this point and said that they bought a used car after they returned home from their honeymoon thanks to generous cash gifts from his mother and Marjorie's parents, a belated wedding present. Marjorie didn't know how to drive and refused to

learn so he was the designated chauffeur, but he didn't mind.

The summer was approaching and a high school chum, Larry, and his girlfriend, Sally, invited Lester and Marjorie for a weekend boating and water skiing at a lake in New Hampshire. "We, of course, accepted the invitation, but neither of us knew how to ski. Larry said it was easy and he would teach us how to launch his boat, captain it in the water, and use skiing safety measures. He said after we both learned how to single and double ski, neither of us would want to get out of the water. He was right. With Larry carefully piloting the boat on the lake, Marjorie was first up. She turned out to be a natural and succeeded on her first attempt on two skis which was quite an accomplishment for a novice," he explained. Lester then paused, frowned, and excused himself to go to the bathroom. I felt like he wanted to avoid describing the rest of the events that weekend, but I wasn't sure why. When he sat back down, I asked him if there was something wrong. He stated he would describe what happened to Marjorie but it would be difficult. I told him to take his time and state anything he wished.

"Later that first afternoon after we all took turns skiing. Near dark, Marjorie asked to go up one more time. I nodded and Larry swung the boat around to take advantage of the remaining sunlight As she had done successfully all day, she got up, this time on one ski, and waved with her free hand and smiled. She was proud of herself. Heck, I wasn't able to single ski at all that day. Then, while we watched from the boat, she went down hard. Larry skillfully turned the boat around towards her and we raised our hands, alerting other boats on the lake Marjorie was in the water. The boat motored directly on the wake of her spill, and she didn't surface. I dove in, thinking her lungs probably were full of water and that she would pop up soon. That didn't happen. Now Larry dove in while Sally steadied the boat. He brought her to

the surface, life jacket intact. I swam over to her. Her face was turning blue and she wasn't moving. We maneuvered her up on the boat and I panicked, calling her name over and over, asking if she was all right. I shook her repeatedly. She was unconscious. Larry, an experienced boatman and a strong swimmer, put her down gently on two large cushions and performed mouth-to-mouth resuscitation. I expected him to revive her and he made several prolonged attempts. But she was gone," Lester said.

I felt a cold rush of despair, stunned. Lester put his head down and cried profusely. Trying to comfort him by putting my hand on his shoulder, he gently pushed it away. "I am so sorry, Lester," I said. He replied, "I know you are." Losing his beautiful wife was devastating and I would later learn this was the first of several tragedies he had to endure with women he loved. Lester got up and walked to his bedroom, limping more noticeably. I gathered my notes and left the apartment, stunned by the tragic event he had just described.

On the short walk home, I tried to gather my thoughts. Lester explained the terrible ordeal clearly and succinctly and, as a result, I gained an insight into his outwardly abrasive demeanor, which appeared to be a mere defense mechanism. However, I hoped that telling about the death of his young wife would prove cathartic.

That night, I tossed and turned, unable to sleep. Lester's mental state was fragile and I didn't want to be responsible for pushing him into further despair. The right thing to do was offer him an out, stopping the interview process. I decided to exercise that option. But I thought it best to wait a few days before I communicated this. Accordingly, I was quite surprised when Lester called the morning after our interview. He said, "Where are you, Grimes. I thought you were coming back today?" We both knew that no such arrangement was made, but knowing Lester, this was his way of telling me he wanted to

continue. We agreed and I walked to his house in the early evening.

We resumed our conversation and Lester appeared relaxed and willing to talk. I felt it was inappropriate to ask him his views on aging and dying because of the circumstances of his wife's death. Instead, I focused on his life thereafter.

Lester stated that after Marjorie's funeral, he thought for days about what he wanted to do and decided he couldn't remain in Bristol. He quit his job at the newspaper and after tearful good-byes to his mom, siblings, and Marjorie's parent's, he got in his car and just drove. "I must have been crazy leaving a good job and my family, but it seemed the right thing to do at the time," he said. He ended up in Bethlehem, Pennsylvania, where he landed a job at Bethlehem Steel in one of their busiest, noisiest factories. Embarking on a move was risky since he had little money, a car needing repair, and no real job prospects. "Finding employment right away was surprising. I was very lucky," Lester said.

At the plant, he learned quickly how to melt and shape steel used in the construction of large buildings and skyscrapers. He worked 12 hour days, 4 days a week in hot, sweaty conditions and was so tired he slept most weekends. "Working long hours kept me out of trouble and I had no social life. I tried to concentrate on work, but Marjorie was constantly on my mind. Soon, I tried to drown my sorrows with booze, but excessive drinking made things worse. I liked my job and didn't want to risk losing it, so I cut down on my drinking. Time went by quickly and before I knew it, two years had passed. Let's see, what happened next....oh yes, John, one of my co-workers invited me to a Christmas party at his house. I only remember a few things about that night. First, the heat wasn't working so the guests huddled around the one fireplace to keep warm. Next, John introduced me to his wife's best friend, Shirley, a stunning divorcee. She was a knockout but I didn't think that pursuing her was a good idea. I was still grieving for Marjorie, but Shirley's kind personality and gentle manner lifted my spirits. She liked me for some reason."

I asked what happened next. Lester replied, "You can probably guess," with a bit of sarcasm in his voice. He was really opening up now. "Well," he continued, "I asked Shirley to go to a company New Year's Party and we danced the night away. She wore a red dress showing lots of cleavage, red high heels, and a pearl necklace. I actually bought a nice blue suit and she couldn't keep her eyes, or hands off me. For the first time in so long, I was happy."

Since the events of the party Lester described in such detail had occurred over 50 years ago, I was impressed with his recall and pleased that Lester's life was turning around for the good at that point. However, I sensed he would reveal more heartache. Turns out, my premonition was correct.

Lester was spent. His demeanor had lightened considerably and I now felt a bond of trust between us. Since he lived alone and made no mention of the current status of his family, I assumed there was a reason. He chose to discuss his life experiences in chronological order.

I put my pen and paper down and leaned forward to say good-bye, but he had fallen asleep. It was safe to assume he wanted to continue our conversation so I wrote a note and placed it on his lap, stating I would return the next day at 10 a.m. and to call me if the day or time was not convenient. I left quietly. I thought about the day's conversation and felt sadness on his behalf. In some ways, he was a depressed, bitter man and was a victim of at least one tragic circumstance – the death of his beloved Marjorie. On the other hand, I saw through his defensive behavior, and underneath was a decent man who couldn't escape his past. He longed for the happiness that had eluded him most of his life.

I anticipated a difficult, emotional final conversation, but Lester seemed up to the task. I asked him the circumstances that brought him to California and the information he provided was both thorough and insightful. He stated that he worked 10 years at Bethlehem Steel, dated Shirley on and off before they married, and had a daughter together, Natalie, who became the "apple of his eye." Sadly, he was diagnosed with bone cancer in 1970. Potent medication diminished the pain, localized in his right leg, but there was no cure. His doctor told him his condition, and the pain, would worsen if he continued the rigors of his job and urged him to pursue a less demanding occupation.

"I was relieved my cancer was treatable, but with a family to support, I was concerned about employment, "Lester stated.

Loving and supportive, Shirley offered an option and called her sister, Meg, in California whose husband, Mark, owned a contracting business in Ventura, north of Los Angeles, specializing in building and installing custom cabinets. Meg was excited about the possibility of having Shirley's family move nearby and knew her husband had been looking to hire another workman since his business was booming. Mark called Lester, knowing he had the manual skills to perform the various shop tasks, and offered him a job. Shirley was elated, but Lester was a bit reluctant to relocate his family. However, after his co-workers at the steel plant threw him a surprise, going-away party, Lester packed up his family and trekked across the country to sunny California.

"While driving, somewhere in New Mexico, I think," he said, "Shirley kept telling me I would love the warm climate and the cool breezes at night off the Pacific Ocean. Good snuggling weather," she insisted. I just smiled and winked into my rear view mirror at little Natalie sitting in the back seat. She smiled and winked back. She was such a cutie. Our trip was a nice adventure,

especially for Natalie, and we enjoyed the sights and sounds of both mountains and desert. We arrived in the dead of night in Ventura and stayed with Meg and Mark for a few weeks until we rented a small two bedroom apartment. They were so helpful."

Lester's mood then darkened and he fell silent. I knew something bad was in the offing. I hesitated and waited for Lester to speak. He then got off the couch, and began pacing in the living room, limping noticeably. He sat down in a few minutes and then bravely described an incredible turn of events. "At Thanksgiving in....well, I don't remember the year, Shirley flew back to Pennsylvania to visit her family. She hadn't seen them in a long time. I promised to take good care of Natalie, now 6 years old, with her sister's help of course." Now tearing and barely audible, he continued as best he could. "

"Shirley was murdered. She was shot outside a restaurant in Bethlehem by her ex-husband while she was walking with her mother to the car," he said. He stopped and looked down.

"I gasped and said," Oh my God. I am so sorry, Lester," which was the second time I offered sincere regrets for his loss; first Marjorie, and now Shirley. At this moment, our conversation had to stop. We both knew that. Lester gathered himself and asked if I could come back in a few days. He said he wanted to talk about his family. I shook his hand, and left.

I arranged a final conversation with Lester for the following week, believing that giving him more time between sessions was necessary. The emotions relating to his painful memories had to be intense. Personally, my stomach was in knots for days. I grieved in my own way for Lester and the loss of the women he loved so much.

Our experience together was a memorable one and our last conversation revealed a grit and determination that I concluded were the roots of Lester's character. Cooperative, very talkative, and in his friendliest mood

yet, he opened up, eagerly responding to all my questions. He explained that following Shirley's death, he was ill-prepared to be a single parent. His beloved Shirley was the rock who kept the family together. He described her as a great wife, mother, cook, and organizer. Now he had to go it alone. Natalie withdrew into a world of darkness and, among other issues, refused to go to school. Weekly therapy had no immediate impact in helping cope with her mother's death. Lester said, "I was mourning for Shirley, but I was determined to do all I could to father and support my daughter through this most difficult time." He went on, referencing the saying, "Time heals all things." He stated that these words were hollow and whoever wrote them never lost a loved one. However, he and Natalie bonded and both somehow endured the nightmare, despite many sleepless nights and a million tears. He knew that their lives had to move forward, but that was easier said than done.

I had now reached an impasse, not knowing what to ask next but much to my relief, Lester kept talking. He described Natalie's upbringing.

"It literally took a village. I employed babysitters, nannies and neighbors. Meg, Shirley's sister, took over much of the time while I worked. Natalie spent many weekends in Ventura with her aunt and uncle and lots of time with them during summer vacation. Meg was a God-send. On one Christmas, Natalie, now a teenager, flew back to visit Shirley's family in Pennsylvania and had a surprise visitor on Christmas Eve, my mother, who had only seen Natalie once before. When Natalie returned home, she talked non-stop about the wonderful time she had. My mom bought her two bags to carry on the airplane to hold the presents she received. Natalie's visit was very special," he stated.

Lester then described his employment after his job with Mark dried up. "I needed money for living expenses, of course, and funds for Natalie's college education. In

1980, I applied for a position at the United States Postal Service in Ventura and luck smiled on me again. I passed the Civil Service test and was offered a job as a Window Clerk. The timing couldn't have been better since Natalie was going to be a junior in high school. During the next two years, I worked full time at the post office and earned a nice wage with benefits. I also worked two part-time jobs on the weekends. I was a working fool but had to do it," he explained.

"I retired from the U.S. Postal Service in 2000 and now receive a great retirement. Thanks to the federal pension I receive and Social Security benefits, my finances are pretty stable. People can say what they want, but Medicare and Social Security are tremendous programs. We old folks have earned these benefits. After all, shouldn't people like me enjoy a slice of the American pie? And now that I think about it, I would have been destitute, broke with nothing if it weren't for Medicare, considering the enormous cost of my cancer treatments and medications. Score that one for Uncle Sam," Lester stated.

Lester then talked about Natalie's life. "She graduated high school with honors and at the ceremony when she spotted me in the stands and waved, I melted. She was the light of my life. I would soon be alone. I never dated and you can probably understand why. I didn't want my heart broken again. Natalie earned a scholarship and with the money I had saved up, she was in good shape financially. After graduating college, she married a very nice young man, John."

He then shared that Natalie and her husband have blessed him with two adorable granddaughters, Shirleen, 10 years old, and Abagail, 8. They live in Goleta, California. John is a banker and does very well. Natalie is a special education aide working part time in a local public school.

"They have a duplex and my granddaughters keep asking me to move into the small unit so they can spend

more time with me. I remain an independent guy and don't want to have to rely on family to care for my needs. That day will come soon enough," Lester explained.

He then leaned back, stretched his legs out, and sighed. Making no mention of aging or death to this point, and I didn't ask, he offered some interesting thoughts. "My life has been a challenge and I have had lots of heartaches, but I know there are many people who are a lot worse off. I read the obituaries every day and think about my own death. You might think this a bit odd, but I have already written my obituary, which I will place in my will. Although I was raised in the Catholic Church, I can't remember the last time I attended mass or confession. I am not a religious man, but I thank God for the hard times I have survived and the will to keep going. I hobble around with a bad leg but at least I have it," he said.

Lester then told me he was very tired. Honestly, listening to and recording his story had exhausted me, too. However, I learned much from him. His courage and determination speak for themselves. Initially, during our conversations, he tried to mask his hurt with sarcasm, but I worked around it because I believed he had a story worth sharing. Deep down, Lester is a softie. I just had to dig and he let me excavate. Sadly, his life was not without misfortune. More than most people experience. But he made the most of every opportunity to create his own happiness and not become a slave to circumstances, however tragic, over which he had no control. In the twilight of his life, he treasures the joy and love Natalie and his grandchildren gift him. That gives him the peace of mind he so richly deserves.

"The oldest trees often bear the sweetest fruit"
-Confucius

Chapter 5 – Haroki (Age 91)

The Veterans residence facility was spacious, well lit, and smelled fresh. The inside walls in the lobby were attractively adorned with colored tiles in a criss-cross design, some inscribed with the name and year of an important battle from the American Revolution to the Gulf War. There was a large living room adjacent to the reception area where several veterans were seated watching ESPN on a large, flat screen T.V. Soft music was playing from several overhead speakers. The décor, including historical scenes painted on cream-colored walls, comfortable couches and chairs, modern lamps, and tables gave the facility an inviting and warm ambiance. The pleasant environment surprised me. The images of dilapidated, dirty, and bug-infested Veterans' facilities, particularly hospitals, I had seen on T.V. news segments and documentary programs flashed in my head. Not here. I introduced myself to the receptionist who offered a friendly hello, and directed me down the east hall to unit 107 where Haroki lived.

Arranged by a friend acquainted with the V.A. Director, I was privy to a few details regarding his participation as a U.S. Army soldier in the 442nd Regimental Combat Team in World War II. This unit was an all-Nisei U.S. Army regiment that served in Europe and, in time, the 442nd became, for its size and length of service, the most decorated unit in U.S. military history.

I expected to be greeted by a frail, aging man, perhaps in a wheel chair. On the contrary, he looked to be

in good physical condition. A man of 91, he could pass for 20 years younger. He was slight of build with piercing brown eyes and a scar on his left cheek.

I extended my hand and he shook it firmly. With a wide grin on his face, he said, "Hi young man." He walked about his unit with ease and possessed a strong presence, exuding a confidence that must have served him well in his soldiering. We sat side by side on his couch, facing each other, and the adventure began. I was very excited to learn about his life and times.

I explained the purpose and content of my book and handed Haroki a copy of the preface. He put on his glasses and read a few paragraphs. "Fortunately, I can still see with the help of these bifocals," he stated. He then asked why I thought his life story would be of interest to readers. The answer was obvious, and I told him that his longevity and participation in World War II as a Japanese-American citizen, no less, were sure to be informative and for many, very inspirational. He nodded, removed his glasses, and stated, "Fair enough, let's get started."

Asking him to provide information concerning his birthplace, education, and family, he was forthcoming and seemed to especially enjoy talking about his sister, Miyako. He was born in Vallejo, California, near San Francisco in 1922 and attended public schools. "My parents were strict, but kind and understanding. Miyako was two years older and always did her best to keep me out of trouble at school and home. My mother, who cleaned day and night to keep a neat and orderly house, expected us to do our share. She often entered our room without warning for an "inspection," as she called them. Miyako stalled her while I threw dirty clothes and school things under my bed. My mother had to know about our little trick, but she didn't let on. I was a little, well, very mischievous, to be honest. But my sister was a gem. She helped me with my homework because I struggled with academics. She was a good sister and tutor," he stated.

"Is she still alive," I inquired. "No, she died young of breast cancer and was only 50," he replied. He explained that her doctors did all they could, but by the time she was diagnosed, the cancer was not treatable and there was nothing they could do. Haroki grieved for a long time and his brother-in-law and Miyako's children were devastated. Her daughter, Chie, never recovered and two years after her mother died, she took her own life. Miyako and Chie's deaths were heartbreaking," he said sadly. I asked if his parents were alive at the time of the Miyako and Chie's death, and he said no; they were spared the agony. Later in our conversation, I would learn more about his father, Katsuro, and mother, Sonomi.

At one point, while we looked at his high school graduation picture, he offered a question of his own.

"Mr. Grimes, what do you think I did after the war?" I shook my head and he chuckled. "I attended the University of Virginia on the G.I. Bill, graduated cum laude, and then taught U.S. History at Jefferson High School in San Francisco. I retired in 1983 with a nice state pension. Along with the federal government benefits through the V.A., I do O.K. financially," he said. I told him that we had several things in common; we taught U.S. History, share a mutual interest in that subject, and are retired educators. He smiled and we again shook hands.

When I inquired about his high school teaching experiences in San Francisco, he recalled fondly that the racial and ethnic diversity of both students and staff made Jefferson High School a unique place. "I was hired by a Black, male principal, the chairman of the History Department was a Hispanic female, and the students I taught were products of diverse backgrounds. We represented a true "melting pot" and teaching and learning was both challenging and engaging. Some of the students, knowing I was a Japanese-American, wanted to

know about my war experiences. I didn't go into detail. Instead, I focused on my family's experiences at Manzanar and the background behind the establishment of the camps. In addition, teaching about the Civil War, I compared the plight of the Japanese-American soldiers with that of the Black slaves who fought for both the North and South. The students were very interested in this comparison and completed some exceptional work – projects, written reports, and oral presentations. Having experienced the events I taught made history come alive. I cherish many wonderful memories with those kids," he said. Haroki's teaching and his personal interest in and commitment to the study of history, personally and academically, added a dimension of authenticity to his story.

We had covered a lot of ground and I asked Haroki if he wanted to end the interview and pick it up again the next day. He said to keep going and after a short break, during which we looked at the second scrapbook, I watched him remove a medal, safely stored in a leather pouch, and hand it to me. I turned the metal piece over to read the inscription that read his rank, name, and unit. This wasn't just any medal. It was the *Medal of Honor*. I was dumbstruck and told him his country owed him a debt of gratitude. I was an honor to be interviewing a true American hero.

Our conversation was going well and the last thing I wanted to do was derail the personal bond we were creating. However, it was time to ask Haroki about the relocation camps. I assumed, and he would soon confirm, that his family was uprooted. By way of background, President Franklin D. Roosevelt signed Executive Order 9066 in 1942, giving the appropriate Military Commander the authority to incarcerate all persons deemed potentially dangerous or disloyal to the United States. Accordingly, in March, 1942, Lieutenant General John DeWitt, head of the Western Defense Command and Fourth Army, issued

the first of 108 military proclamations that resulted in the forced relocation to guarded camps of more than 110,000 people of Japanese ancestry on the West Coast. The majority were U.S. citizens.

I asked, "When was your family relocated?" Hesitating slightly, Haroki nodded. He then was silent for a few minutes. This pause was uncomfortable, but he soon opened up. Unlike previous positive, upbeat responses, he offered comments stinging with contempt. Consequently, I now felt more like a journalist than an author. Understanding that providing details of his family's relocation had to be painful, I transcribed his words as stated and didn't ask him to elaborate on any of the questions. Respecting his feelings was paramount.

He said," The Japanese people living on the west coast were embarrassed. No, that's the wrong word. We were humiliated when the attack on Pearl Harbor took place, but few believed that event would result in taking away our homes or our rights. We were American citizens, after all. The government gave Japanese-Americans little time to pack up and prepare to move. My family boarded a bus on May 1, 1942, taking all detainees to Manzanar at the foot of the Sierra Nevada Mountains. I remember that day as if it were yesterday."

I then asked, "What were the conditions like there?" His reply was brief and descriptive. "Horrific. The housing units were small, poorly lit with no heat, and no indoor plumbing. The outhouses were dirty and the smell was putrid. It was a glorified prison and an uncertain of future was a constant worry. That created stress, but our people were cooperative – some would say, passive. I couldn't believe I was actually there." I asked, "Were you angry?" "No," he responded. "I was frustrated and like a lot of my contemporaries in the camp, I wanted to prove my loyalty to America. We knew that the only way to do that was to enlist, but it took time until the government made it happen."

My research revealed that in 1943 the U.S. government reversed its previous decision on Japanese-Americans serving in the military and approved the formation of a Japanese-American combat unit. Shortly thereafter, the government required that all internees answer a loyalty questionnaire, which was used to register the Nisei for the draft. Haroki was part of the 75% answering that they were willing to enlist and swear allegiance to the United States. Months later, he boarded another bus, this time taking him to Oakland, California, for processing and training. He stated, "Leaving my family was very difficult, but I had a lot to prove to myself and the country I still loved." He became a pioneer member of the 442nd Regiment.

The interview had reached a logical stopping point so I suggested we continue another day. Hiroki was understandably tired and asked that I call him to schedule another meeting. I walked to my car and thought about the contrasting roles Charles, (Chapter 1) Jakub, (Chapter 3) and Haroki had played during World War II. Charles was stationed in a location far removed from combat and Jakub, a civilian, performed vital tasks in research and aircraft design in complete safety. Although I was yet to learn specifics about his combat experiences, it was a given he was often in harm's way, evidenced by his receipt of the prestigious *Medal of Honor*. The irony here is that he was interred for a year before he was permitted to enlist, and then risked his life fighting for a country that had nearly stripped him of his dignity and self-respect. His service, and that of his military colleagues, was a testament to determination, persistence, bravery, and loyalty. I wondered to what extent he would share his experiences in battle.

A week later on a warm, sunny day I met Haroki outside on the V.A. patio courtyard for our second encounter. He was in good spirits and seemed anxious to talk. Turns out, it was not about the war. Before I could

ask a question, he started talking. "I have given considerable thought about my family and want to tell you more about them," he said. "Please do," I replied.

The next hour he provided many details about his father, mother and sister. His manner and voice were melancholy and reflected memories that were both pleasant and sad. He stated his parents were born in Honshu Province, Japan, and immigrated to America a year after they married. His father couldn't make a living as a fisherman and dreamed of a better life in America. They booked tickets on a freighter that docked in San Francisco in 1918. The voyage was rough and especially uncomfortable for his mother pregnant with his sister. The couple settled in Vallejo and lived with his father's brother, Koichi, a Protestant minister, until they earned enough money to buy a house. Koichi baptized each family member. Haroki said, "I remember attending church every Sunday. Miyako and I were raised with Christian values which remain important in my life today."

I asked Haroki about his parents after the war. He stated that they managed to endure Manzanar the best they could. They were released a month after the Japanese surrendered to the Allies on September 2, 1945. Much to their surprise, when they returned home their house was in good condition. No one lived there during their absence and they retained ownership. However, the experience at Manzanar irreparably damaged his father's spirit. He died in 1950 at the age of 57. Distraught without her loving husband, his mother died a year later after an extended bout with Pneumonia.

Haroki continued, but his voice softened and demeanor turned somber. "My immediate family has passed and I am the sole survivor. By all rights, I should have been killed in the war. But, for good or bad, I am still here. My faith has kept me strong. I know I will see my family again in heaven."

His description about his unlikely survival against the premature death of his sister and the passing of his parents is understandable. Reasoning when and why death occurs is as problematic as it is unpredictable. I am reminded of a passage from Philippians 4:7 - "The peace of God, which transcends all understanding, will guard your hearts and minds in Jesus Christ." Haroki acknowledged the power of these words.

I asked him if he ever remarried.

"No, I did not. Do you think it is too late?" he retorted. I told him it was never too late. The levity broke the ice, however abbreviated. Maintaining the light, humorous tone, he asked me if there was a hot female I could fix him up with. We both laughed. "Seriously," he said, "I never really looked to get married. I am not afraid of a commitment, but didn't meet anyone who captured my heart. Perhaps the war soured me. I did have a few opportunities, though. When I taught high school a very attractive teaching colleague used to chase me down the hall, but she never caught up with me; I was too fast – you know, my military training and all. We were just friends."

Haroki excused himself to return to his apartment, perhaps to retrieve one of his scrapbooks, but he didn't say. While he was gone, I thought about what might have been going through his mind. Having returned from war alive, men often declined to talk about their experiences. The sheer horror of combat, seeing fellow soldiers maimed or killed in the worst possible circumstances can puncture and paralyze the minds of even the most stable men. That said, I was prepared to accept the possibility that he wouldn't want to share his travails. But he did.

He sat down and handed me a can of Coke. In response to a question about his military training after enlistment, he provided an abundance of information, so much so that I had to ask him to repeat several of his recollections. One such memory opened my olfactory. He leapfrogged my question and said, "I will never forget the

smell of exposed flesh and the nausea I felt. In one fire fight two of my closest buddies were saturated by a German flame thrower, and I could do nothing to save them. I was overcome by the stench of their burns and watched them incinerate. I threw up all over myself."

This image impacted me in a most disturbing way, but I appreciated his honest account. He went on to say that watching his friends die had aged him. He then produced two photographs of himself from an envelope he placed in one of his scrapbooks. One was taken the day he arrived In Oakland for processing and the other in 1945 after his discharge. The first picture showed a youthful man, 22 years old. In the other picture, he had aged noticeably and looked 10 years older. These photographs evidence the physical toll the war had on him. The differences were striking.

Hiroki said, "I am sorry, Mr. Grimes. You asked a question before. What was it?" "It concerned your military training," I answered.

"Oh yes, my training. It was tough, very tough. Understand, despite the oath of allegiance we took, the officers and drill instructors didn't trust us. Why would they trust Nisei? We were not just "Japs," as they called us. We were symbols of the death and destruction at Pearl Harbor. The D.I.'s did all they could to make us fail. But we were strong and to the best of my knowledge, no one in our regiment washed out. We were determined."

I told Haroki I learned his regiment moved quickly and fought bravely in Europe. He stated, "In less than a year, our unit fought in Italy, France, and Germany. Battles were ferocious, particularly in Germany and the fighting was often hand-to-hand. Their soldiers fought with desperation because they were losing the war. We suffered many casualties. I had to be alert at all times because I never knew if I was in the sights of an enemy sniper. Night was especially eerie and a few times the enemy was only a few meters away. I was fortunate to be

fighting with a group of brave and skilled soldiers. But don't think for a minute that we weren't scared. Well, terrified would be a better word."

Naively, I asked him when he was able to sleep. He chuckled, leaned back and volleyed back a sarcastic response. "Almost never," he said. "We used the buddy system and when possible we got a little shut eye, but with only one eye closed. That is the truth my friend." He then stated that sleep was almost always interrupted by the sound of artillery or bombs in the distance or rifle fire at close range. He and his comrades lived and fought in a constant state of fatigue but somehow they just kept going. Recalling one rare exception, he stated there was a period of three consecutive days, he thought in France, where there was no shelling, no fighting, and no killing.

Haroki was both informative and descriptive during our conversations. He was a product of a loving family, but their premature death deeply saddened him. A simple, decent, and honest man, his service in defense of our country was beyond the call of duty. Although he referred to the Japanese-American people as passive, the young Nisei who fought and died in Europe were anything but. Like many fellow soldiers, he demonstrated a quiet resolve to weather the storm of internment, survive the brutality of combat, and rebuild his life after the war. He is a survivor and his spirit to live on is unshakable. The war aged him, understandably so, but he remains a monument to longevity. His response to my final question was telling. I asked, "You were close to death many times, yet you survived. Why?" He replied, "It wasn't my time. God's purpose for my life had not yet been fulfilled." I shook his hand and told him I was privileged to know a true American hero and write his story.

"We are here to laugh at the odds and live our lives so well that death will tremble to take us"
-Charles Bukowski

Chapter 6 – Simone (Age 75)

Simone is an intelligent, spunky, beautiful African-American woman whose presence lights up a room. Her charismatic nature and natural charm showcase a caring, affirming personality. I met her randomly at a social mixer at a Health Care Center in Santa Clarita, California, where I was recruiting seniors to interview for my book. Striving for diversity in the text, I sought a female of color who could provide a compelling saga. Suddenly, I discovered Simone, or should I say, she discovered me. When she learned I was writing a book about aging, she shouted, "You definitely want me in it." That would remain to be seen, but I sensed she might have a fascinating life story to tell. A brief conversation with her convinced me I had stumbled onto a woman whose life experiences would be of great interest to readers.

I wanted to meet soon, but she had to check her calendar. Apparently, Simone was very active. We spoke a few days later and she stated she had bridge club on Monday and Pilates on Tuesday and Thursday. Each Wednesday was movie day at the health center. Time spent exercising and socializing had to surpass most people her age, but her chosen activities were a personal priority, and deservedly so. We settled for the coming Friday, but Simone threw me a curve. Normally, for convenience sake, I arrange interviews at the residence facility of the senior, but much to my surprise she asked to

meet her at the city public library. In order for us to talk freely, she reserved a private, soundproof room. She was a take-charge woman. When I arrived, she was already in the conference room and had several notebooks, manila folders, and books on the table in front of her with papers scattered about, much like one would expect of a student. Turns out, she *was* a student. She gave me a warm greeting and motioned for me to sit down. I asked her about the materials on the table. She stated, "I put two wonderful children through college. I have no regrets in that regard. Angela and Raven are making a difference in the world. But now it's my turn. I'm attending a community college in my fourth semester and plan to enroll at a public four-year university next fall. My goal is to earn a B.A. Degree in Economics. Now, what do you think about that?" she asked, cocking her head to the side, smiling.

I replied, "I think it's great." My, this woman is a bundle of energy and ambitious, too. Attending college at age 75 is a testament to her determination and youthful spirit. Her behavior reflected great resolve, and I had no doubt she would achieve her educational goal. Wild horses couldn't stop her.

Then, we got down to business, and I started the interview with a question about the father of the girls.

"My husband, Willie, died of cancer when the twins were young," she said. "He was only 52 years old and at the time of his death, he was the sole bread winner. I was a housewife. Rough times were ahead. I worked two jobs and a special nanny cared for the girls in my absence. We managed to stay afloat, but barely. Fortunately, Macon – that's in Georgia, was kid-friendly and the public schools were excellent, at least at that time. I grieved for Willie a long time as did my twin daughters, but I kept busy working and, as time passed, the pain lessened. I still think about him every day. He was a shy, quiet man. As you probably can imagine, we were definite opposites. Our

daughters, families and friends appreciated his kind and gentle manner. I loved him so."

I replied, "Did you ever remarry?" "I had many offers, but didn't believe it fair to Angela and Raven. The bond with their father was strong although they were only 7 years old at the time of his death. Years later my friends, as they had done every so often, encouraged me to date. I did, but Willie remains tucked inside my heart and I won't make room for another," she stated.

I asked Simone to describe her childhood and upbringing. She was born in Macon, Georgia, in 1938 to loving, religious parents. She was the middle child with an older brother, Malcolm, and a younger sister, Diana. Her father was a Baptist preacher who ministered to a large, predominantly Black congregation. "Attending church twice a week, reading the Bible, and holding family first in our hearts and minds were all expectations of my father and mother. They were wonderful parents and shaped the values that still guide me today," she said.

"My brother, sister, and I liked school and each of us excelled in different ways. Malcolm was an average student but was a three-sport letterman in high school. He still holds the Georgia state track record in the 100 meter sprint. Sister Diana was a social butterfly all through her school years and was prom queen her senior year. She worked hard and became an excellent student, earning an academic college scholarship. I earned a "B" average and participated on the debate team and was captain of the chess club. I guess I was a bit of a nerd."

I paused, my mind swimming with questions for Simone, one of which I put at the top of the list. Taken by her flirtatious demeanor, I inquired," Simone, you look and act younger than your age. What's your secret?"

She replied, "You flatter me, Mr. Grimes. Thank you but I have no secrets. I suppose exercising, eating healthy, and staying busy have contributed to a good life. Frankly, I don't give a lot of thought to aging. It may

sound like a cliché – well, it is, but I live one day at a time and am blessed I wake up every morning a happy woman. My Christian faith continues to give me strength and purpose."

I responded, asking "What do you believe to be your purpose?" "Good question," she said. "Glorifying God all ways possible and devoting my time and energy to raising two exceptional daughters. They light my life. Now that I think about it, I don't take things too seriously as far as my own wants and desires are concerned. I look beyond earthly thoughts and actions as Jesus taught. Many passages in the scriptures confirm God's intent to provide what we need, but for each of us to seek the gift of salvation. I have led a long life, but it can end at any time. I want to take advantage of every minute." I then commented, "Your words reflect an urgency to live a life with conviction and passion. Good for you!"

We had reached a logical stopping point and when I suggested we either take a break or continue our dialogue another time, Simone asked that we meet again the next Friday. Typical of a conscientious student, she had a paper to write and a test in her science class to study for and needed to work on those tasks in the conference room for a few hours. I thanked her and wished her well.

Driving home, I ruminated about the interview with Simone. She was very verbal and expressed herself clearly, more articulate and replete in details than any of the seniors with whom I had previously spoken. She had a good sense of herself and a personality bubbling with confidence and optimism. Before I left, she provided a preview of what would prove to be a highly interesting next session. "My great-great grandfather was a slave, escaped from a brutal master, and eventually fought for the North in the Civil War. His life was amazing." I couldn't wait to hear all about this man.

I arrived at the appointed time a week later and, as I anticipated, Simone was hard at work in the same

conference room. I initiated a hug and I asked about the paper she was writing the last time we met and how she did on the science test. "Oh, thanks for asking. I turned in the paper but I won't get it back until next week. But I aced the science test." She evidently was well versed on colloquial expressions. Most seniors wouldn't know, let alone use, phrases like, "aced the test." I replied, "Good job. What are you working on now?" I asked. "Another paper," she stated. "However, this time I have to submit it online. I am learning to use technology. I have been a pencil and paper gal my entire life so modern technology is a bit scary, but once you get the hang of it, it is fun," she commented.

Although I was looking forward to hearing about Simone's great-great grandfather, I decided to inquire further about her family and led with a question about her daughters – where they were and what they were doing. She stated, "O.K. Angela and Raven had successful high school experiences and both attended the University of Tennessee in Knoxville on basketball scholarships. For good or bad, they grew up dressing, thinking, and acting alike, and were practically inseparable. When they were born, my pediatrician told Willie and me to read up on twins. He said twins were a gift from God, but providing for their unique needs and adjusting to their natural inclination to be together would be challenging. He said it was all about genetics. After raising them as a single mother during their formative years, I learned that the doctor was correct. They both live and work in Oxnard, not too far from here. Angela is an elementary school teacher and coaches the Girls Varsity Basketball team at one of the best high schools in the area. Raven is the Director of the Recreation Department which is a very responsible job. Both girls are married and I have great sons-in-law. The girls have blessed me with four grandchildren, two boys and two girls. Their ages range

from 10 to 18. They love me to pieces, and the feeling is mutual.

"What do they call you," I inquired. She laughed out loud and said, "Si" with a long "i." When they were babies learning to talk, I kept repeating my name while changing their diapers or bathing them. I didn't want to be called grandma. That term has no pizzazz. Besides, it makes me feel old. None of the children could say the last syllable of my name, so "Si" has stuck, and that's fine with me. Actually, I think it's kind of a cute name, don't you think?" I nodded.

After a break, Simone and I settled into a most intriguing conversation about her great-great grandfather, Lucius. She said her distant families on both sides had kept track of his adventures as a young plantation slave outside Atlanta, his stint in the Union Army during the Civil War, and his life after the war. Interestingly, Simone was in possession of a picture of her great-great grandfather and two letters received by his older sister, a home slave in South Carolina, before and during the war. She opened a manila folder and put the picture in front of me. I examined it and was surprised that it was in good condition – black and white, of course. Simone identified Lucius standing on the far left. He was a tall, burly man and had sergeant stripes on his uniform sleeves. Accordingly, she believed he must have been an able leader and a courageous soldier. At this point, I wondered how Lucius' sister, living in the Confederate state of South Carolina, managed to receive the letters. More on that later.

Before removing the letters from the envelope, she remarked that she doubted Lucius could read or write and believed both letters must have been written by a fellow soldier who was somewhat educated. Lucius probably dictated. Simone pushed the letters towards me so I could read them. Both were legible, and written on paper that had turned yellow. By the positioning of the letters and the

dark stain, the writing implement was probably a quill pen. With no lines to guide the unknown writer, the words were carefully written across with appropriate spacing. One statement of interest concerned Lucius' frustration being assigned manual labor and cooking duties. His commanding officer was white and the harsh treatment to which the black soldiers were subjected made him feel like a slave again. This was terrible, but he had to endure it somehow. After all, the white and black soldiers were fighting on the same side.

A portion of one of the letters read, *"The officers are against us and beat us because we are Negroes. They call us terrible names and we have to take it. If we quarrel with them, they will shoot us. It is best to keep quiet and do what they tell us. I thought we be treated with respect but they give us no dignity. We were loyal soldiers. It took a long time before they let us fight. When we did, we killed a lot of Rebs."*

Simone stated," There is a journal that was kept by Lucius' mother which recorded the circumstances of his life after the war. However, the journal was lost. So details about that period of his life are just word-of-mouth. I understand, though, that Lucius settled in Boston after the war, married, and had two children. Lacking a formal education, he worked at a livery stable and remained there for many years. His boss must have appreciated his strength, body size, and ability to work whatever hours were required. After spending long, hot days on the plantation, working in the livery stable had to be a gift."

I was curious about how the letters were secured by Jerome's sister since she was living in a belligerent Southern state. The Confederates were certainly not going to deliver mail from the north. Simone said that one of the relatively unknown tasks performed by the *Underground Railroad*, besides ushering slaves secretly out of the South, was to deliver letters when the whereabouts of the recipients was known and the conditions safe. This

practice was not a regular routine and obviously very dangerous.

There are a number of genealogy websites that trace family lineage and history, and I asked Simone if she had accessed any. She said she had not. I offered to help as my interest intensified about her great-great grandfather's life. He had to be a fascinating man. A few days after the interview, I conducted research on an authoritative genealogy website in the hopes of learning more about Simone's family, and Lucius in particular. There weren't many details to be had, but I accessed a record of his death certificate through the Registry Division of the city of Boston stating that Lucius Quincy Brown died on September 18, 1893, in Boston, Massachusetts. The cause of death was not given. Simone stated he was a young man, perhaps in his early 30s when he escaped the plantation in Georgia. If my math is correct, he lived into his early 60s. Statistics on longevity in America indicate the average lifespan of a male born around 1830 was 45 years. Consequently, Lucius' age at the time of his death far exceeded that number. Simone's paternal family had good genes. Her age, spirit, and personal durability validate the genetics.

Simone's family lineage could be traced nearly 200 years and beginning with her great great-great grandfather, longevity appeared to be a predominant family characteristic. I explored this and asked Simone how long her parents lived. "My mother died in her sleep at age 95 just 5 years ago. My father died of lung cancer at age 91. My grandparents also lived well into their 90s. My parents were a great couple and terrific parents. They loved each other dearly and they adored us kids. Growing up, none of us got away with anything though. Preachers' kids have a reputation of being wild, but our parents controlled us pretty well. They worked together in managing our behavior and we couldn't play one against the other, as many kids do. But it wasn't for lack of trying." We chuckled simultaneously. Simone stated earlier that her values, taught and modeled by her parents, remained intact throughout her life and believed that she had passed those qualities on to her own kids.

During both interviews, it became apparent she had lived a good life and was aging well, and slowly, both physically and mentally. Her active lifestyle, pursuit of a college degree, as well as living close to her kids and grandchildren, keeps her vibrant and happy. The longevity of her parents and grandparents evidences sturdy genes. Barring something unforeseen, she was likely to equal or exceed the ages of her family elders.

Simone is a kind, loving, and deeply religious woman. Her compassion, commitment to furthering her education, and love of family coincide; in fact, complement her spiritual convictions. She possesses a depth of character and an abiding faith in God. That said, I was compelled to ask about her views on death and the afterlife.

I opened with this question. "What are your thoughts on death and the afterlife?" Her answer typified her ability to recall details from her life long ago while infusing a little humor.

"Death is the great equalizer and humbles us all – no matter your age or station in life. We enter the world alone and take what the Lord gives us. When we die, our souls journey with us. The only difference is that when we leave we take our soul with us," she said.

I countered, "What is and where is heaven?" She referenced again her father was a preacher, but he didn't confine his knowledge and belief in the scriptures to his flock.

Simone said, "At supper time, my brother, sister, and I often posed questions about his sermons. Honestly, we didn't always understand the message spoken at church that day and asked him to explain. He clarified in language we understood. However, he took forever to

deliver it because he invariably answered our questions by asking his own. My father was a Biblical scholar, and he had a colorful personality – always teaching. My mother told us that was why he was so popular with his congregation. Anyway, I didn't answer your question yet….forgive me, I am getting to it."

"No worries, this is interesting stuff, "I said.

She said heaven was a topic often discussed at supper and that her father would tell them to go get their Bibles and read up on it. Her brother, Malcolm, felt very frustrated with their father's tactic of avoidance. "He didn't like it when his math teacher failed to give an answer to a thought problem, wanting students to do the "work" first," she said. "Our father did the same thing. "As you can probably tell, meal time was always lively with stimulating conversation," Simone explained.

Still curious about her views on heaven, Simone offered a few Biblical references. "The books of Romans, Luke, and Mark contained passages about heaven and eternity, but the one that sticks with me is 1 John 5, chapter 13. It reads something like this. "*Believe in the name of the Son of God that you may have eternal life.*" I know that God welcomes us to heaven based on our faith and good works. Is heaven a place? Yes, it houses our spirit. However, we mortals cannot possibly have a complete understanding of heaven but I plan to join my husband there," she said.

We looked at each other, smiling, and realized our time together had come to an end. Simone's drive, energy, devotion to God and family, and the educational goals to which she aspires give her a special status in my eyes. No couch potato, she is a woman of action. An exceptional person, I have been privileged to have been the recipient of a life story full of warmth, good will, optimism, and an accounting of a most fascinating family history. But she isn't done yet!

"I don't feel old. I don't feel anything until noon.
Then it's time for my nap"
-Bob Hope

Chapter 7 – Angelica (Age 82)

The words he spoke while sitting on a park bench convey exactly how I feel when interviewing an individual about to tell a life story. "Life is a box of chocolates. You never know what you're going to get," Forrest Gump said in the movie of the same name. So true. My first priority is to determine if experiences shared by seniors will be of compelling interest to readers. Accordingly, my selection instincts must be keen in determining which seniors are featured in their own chapter. After listening for just a few minutes to what she had to say, I had no doubt that Angelica fit my personal criteria. At the conclusion of our initial conversation – some 3 ½ hours later, she said there was much more to tell, particularly about life events during World War II and her battles with cancer. I drove home looking forward to learning more, anticipating that her story would encompass a complete chapter. Turns out, an entire book on her life would be more like it.

In most interviews there is give and take: questions, answers, follow-up question I record in my notepad. But when I asked Angelica to talk about her life, she took the ball and ran with it. She first described her current activities, rather than offering biographical information in chronological order, which was the typical pattern. She took charge and began to share her story without interruption. Consequently, I locked in automatic pilot and enjoyed the ride. Admittedly, I was somewhat

surprised, but impressed, that she considered herself a *techy*. She had purchased an Apple P.C. 20 years ago and has been using a computer of one kind or another ever since. I learned in our subsequent meeting she has an iMac Computer, an iPod with Bose ear phones, and an iPhone which she plans to trade in for the new iPhone 5c. She said the new model has a much better camera and that no password was needed because it activates by reading the users' fingerprints. Who knew? Her knowledge and application of technology is incredible. Angelica just might be one of a kind that way. Further evidencing her technological prowess, in our phone conversation to schedule the first interview, she stated that she had to check her electronic calendar to see when she was free. I suspect that a very small percentage of seniors her age use a computer or other electronic devices with such skill and frequency.

Angelica led with a personal endorsement of volunteerism evidenced by her participation in *Habitat for Humanity*. She stated, "I am a board member of the organization and help oversee home sales in the Santa Barbara area." She described in detail the process by which interested individuals apply, qualify, and purchase. Successful applicants own the property and the mortgage is interest-free. I was surprised to learn the board of directors, not banks, establish prices and collect mortgage payments. Circumventing red tape and the anxiety normally associated with home purchases makes the process run smoothly. Angelica provides information to applicants and is available to help educate all interested parties including the many non-English speaking families.

Angelica then shared information about her involvement in another activity and her words took on a very personal dimension.

"I am on the board of directors of a non-profit foundation, *Freedom to Choose*, the service arm of the University of Santa Monica." A husband and wife team of

the university facilitates a three day workshop at the Maximum Security Women's Prison in Chowchilla, California, twice a year. Seventy or eighty volunteers, including Angelica, all graduates of the university's master's degree program, travel at their own expense to assist facilitating the workshops. The emphasis in the sessions is grounded on a loving, non-judgmental premise, and the women respond well, often in a most demonstrably emotional way. Angelica has endeared herself to the inmates. They call her *grandma rock* and it is easy to understand why.

Angelica is very proud of the great work the volunteers do encouraging the female inmates. She said that a documentary on the workshops was made several years ago and that it received an award at the Cannes Film Festival in France. She and her fellow volunteers are making a significant difference in the lives of many women, giving each a renewed sense of hope for the future.

Born in Brooklyn, New York, in 1931, during the *Great Depression*, Angelica was a product of a diverse family. Her father, a Russian Jew and a plumber by trade, had twelve siblings with various religious affiliations: traditional Jews, a Christian Scientist, one Catholic, and six Jesus Jews. Her mother was Swedish and Angelica described her as mean-spirited. The two were estranged most of Angelica's life. "When I tried to hug her, she asked me what I wanted." Sad indeed. Consequently, she gravitated to her paternal grandfather.

"He shaped my life. He was a loving, kind, compassionate man and taught me arithmetic on the run while shopping together at the neighborhood delicatessen. When he was sick, I skipped school and picked flowers for him. When I arrived at his tenement with a bouquet, he was happy to see me, but asked what I was doing out of school. He smiled just the same." Her grandfather readily accepted her love and was always the protector. However,

Angelica said her life changed, not for good, when he moved to Indiana. He stabilized her life in so many ways for so long and she felt empty when he moved.

When Angelica offered more information about her childhood, I noticed a hummingbird helping himself at the feeder mounted outside on the patio above us, adjacent to her living room window. She recognized the little guy with a beautiful red chest, and said that one day while reading outside, he flitted up to the feeder and she asked him to wing over and say hello. He flew over close to her face as requested. It was obvious Angelica had a deep connection with nature. Throughout the rest of our conversation, other hummingbirds fed at the spout, and Angelica identified one with a black chest as territorial, often chasing his neighborhood friends away from *his* feeder. Funny! There was something mystical about the appearance of the hummingbirds, which fed often there, and turned to face and Angelica while still fluttering their tiny wings. She spoke to them affectionately, like a parent to a child, and they seemed to understand.

Without hesitating, Angelica described her work history. She said she has always worked. Her first job was at age 12 in a factory in Brooklyn, earning $24 a week. "My father took $19 and I was left with $5. I didn't like my job, but I learned two things quickly. First, I vowed never to work in a factory again (and she didn't), and that in the future I would keep $19 and give my father $5 (and she did)." Other jobs she held included clerking at F.W. Woolworth after school and when she was older, and managing real estate for an investor in Manhattan. She explained, "I helped integrate housing in New York City and that took some courage. In fact, when I arranged for a nice African-American couple to rent an apartment, my life was threatened. The fact that no landlord, except for my boss, rented to Blacks was unconscionable. I feel good knowing I helped open up housing opportunities for minorities." She went on to say that while still living in

New York, she worked at a men's clothing store. When I asked her why, she stated, "To meet men, of course."

I wondered about Angelica's family and she must have read my mind. She spoke extensively about them, offering details of the lives of her son, Gary, 50, daughter Amanda, 48, and her husband, Marty, now deceased.

Angelica said, "Hospitals are for sick people, so both children were born at home. I insisted on that. The children grew up healthy and happy. But Gary has Stargardt disease, a genetic vision disorder, and is nearly blind. My son is a good man; very intelligent. He earned a Bachelor's degree from UCSB in Religious Studies and later received a Master's Degree in Transpersonal Psychology. Gary has never come to terms with his blindness and when he was growing up I refused to enable him. Rather, I used *tough love* when we lived in Florida. I forced him to use public transportation and he quickly learned to get around. He now lives in New York and travels the subways anywhere in the city with ease." Angelica added her son has excellent paternal instincts and was a great stay-at-home dad for his two children for 11 years. He is now divorced.

Angelica's daughter, Amanda, lives in Decatur, Georgia, and is divorced with one child. Like her brother, she is very intelligent. She earned a Bachelor of Arts degree in Clinical Nutrition from CSUN and a Master's Degree in the same subject from NYU.

"She is the kindest woman I know. One day around Thanksgiving, leading a project for Heartfelt Foundation at a day center on skid row in Los Angeles, I brought a full Thanksgiving Dinner, clothing, shoes, and other items to distribute. Amanda, 14-years-old at that time, accompanied me and served juice to men waiting in line for dinner. A few minutes passed and I noticed she was asking a homeless woman with no shoes and bloody feet to try on a new pair of shoes at a vendor's enclosure. She sat the woman down, washed her feet, and helped fit

her with shoes. I approached this Biblical encounter, shook my head, smiled, and thought to myself, who does this? Amanda had done an incredibly good deed, and frankly, I wasn't surprised." Even recently, Angelica noted that Amanda had flown out to help organize her apartment. She cleaned, put things away, and resurfaced the deck on the patio. Amanda's actions, then and now, evidence a strong family value of humanity and good will to others.

It's apparent that Angelica, her grandfather, and her adult children share common characteristics: devotion to family, and unselfish service to others. More information about the humanitarian role Angelica's grandfather played to help immigrants is forthcoming. For now, though, the first interview is complete. I thoroughly enjoyed the conversation and told Angelica I would contact her to arrange a follow-up visit.

Our next interview, a week later, was as intriguing as the first, maybe more so. Angelica began by sharing that a girlfriend introduced her to her future husband, Marty, at a social function in New York, and they hit it off immediately.

"He was a handsome, musically talented Jewish man; a trumpeter who played for several big bands in many different venues. Due to his preference for a warmer climate and for working on a more consistent basis, we eventually moved to Hollywood, Florida. Marty was a dyed-in-the-wool bachelor, and since I was not an advocate for marriage anyway, our relationship had a strong foundation. We decided to live together, a social taboo in those days. But we decided that was the right thing to do." Backing up a bit in time, she said that Marty was her 3rd husband and that she didn't do very well with marriage. She stated they married before the children were old enough to attend school, not wishing to stigmatize them. She knew classmates would make fun of them and there was no reason to put either child through

that. She then shared a very touching moment regarding a gift Marty provided at the birth of their daughter, Amanda. She stated, "I told you previously that both children were born at home. When Amanda came into the world, the doctor had not yet arrived so with umbilical cord still attached, Marty performed midwife duties and put a blanket around our precious baby and nursed her with his pinkie finger until I could breast feed. I will not forget the look on his face. He was a proud father, and at that moment, I could not have loved him more."

She then shared that years later the two divorced and soon after Marty contracted pancreatic cancer. He moved back to New York and the children were with him there until he died. Amanda told her mother that her father was the first to touch her when she was born and she was the last person to reciprocate as he died, a heart-felt rendition of the unique bond between Marty and his precious Amanda, their lives having gone full circle.

She celebrated the wonderful things her grandfather had done on behalf of his fellow man. At the turn of the century, immigrants to America flooded Ellis Island in New York with no identification papers. Without the proper documents, many were turned away and sent home. Although he had twelve children of his own, all living in a small apartment, he felt a need to help people he didn't know acclimate to their new life in America. He went to the docks and intervened on their behalf with the U.S. Immigration Authority, coaxing officials to allow immigrants to enter. Angelica didn't know if money was exchanged in the process, but she said he vouched for many families and personally took them in until they could find work and a place to live. "Fortunately," she said, "My grandfather owned a business, sewing uniforms for the United States government and in doing so he gained an advantage in helping out the poor immigrants who were in no position to help themselves. He was a remarkable man."

Before recounting Angelica's experiences at home during World War II and her battle with two forms of cancer, I offer a few thoughts on her spirituality.

In her words, "My life is blessed. I live on Social Security, have traveled overseas, and earned good money during the many years of my employment, which I spent freely. I never feel poor and pay my own bills." Now she watches life and enjoys doing so and, as with her hummingbird friends, she is in tune with nature like never before. Then, for some reason and out of the blue, she recalled a brief dialogue in the movie, *Oh God*, in which John Denver (Jerry) and George Burns (God) exchanged a bit of levity. Denver is driving his car and God's voice is heard on the radio, "I want you to carry my message to the people; no one is listening to me." Denver replies, "God, why me, I am not religious." God replies, "Neither am I." Angelica relates to the content of their exchange. In talking with her, including our final conversation, it was apparent that she held close to her convictions, spiritual and religious, and she recognized the importance of both, blending them together to establish a tranquility of mind and spirit.

During World War II, Americans at home made varying contributions to the war effort to enhance morale. Angelica described one such activity. "I was 14 or 15 years old when the war was heating up, and my older sister and a girlfriend, who dated only sailors, cased out the good looking guys in uniform on Coney Island." But Angelica took it one step further and adopted a ward at a Naval Hospital by visiting the injured. She remembers one sailor who had his leg amputated asked her if she could get him a beer. True to form, Angelica smuggled one in for him. In addition, Angelica's mom and dad hosted parties on weekends and made sure there was one young lady for each sailor. As you can see, Angelica's family did a world of good for the young men in uniform, making them feel at home, valued, and loved.

In the final phase of our interview we discussed Angelica's health status, specifically her bouts with two types of cancer, and later her personal philosophy about life. The confidence in her words revealed a strong resilience and a commitment to fight and defeat the toxic, life-threatening cancers.

"At age 30, I was diagnosed with uterine cancer and was told by an oncologist that I had only a 25% chance of survival." Demonstrating strength of character, she countered this threat by utilizing the advice of a spiritual teacher. As the student, she became a health nut, altering immediately her food and life behaviors. Much to her credit and that of her teacher, she beat the cancer and without the use of traditional medical treatments. She then described her next fight, this time with lung cancer, diagnosed 46 years later.

"A biopsy showed cancerous cells in my lungs, but I was determined to enhance my immune system to fight off the danger," she said. She received treatment from a traditional Chinese doctor and used herbs prescribed for one year. Despite slight improvement, surgery was necessary and half her left lung was removed. Interestingly, she now uses regular medicine when necessary. A cancer survivor, not once, but twice, she now believed it was time for a change in her mental perspective, and looked to a higher power.

With conviction in her voice, the words stirred my senses. She stated she was a divine being having a human experience, and is certain she doesn't have to die to go to heaven. Explaining, she stated, "A person can peel off layers of conditioning, if so inclined, and experience a true self." She concluded by referencing a conversation in which God told her she would live until she was 90. With much soul searching and through divine inspiration, she has reconciled her life.

Angelica possesses many gifts and continues to make the world a better place. Her grandfather modeled

selfless humanity and she mirrors his efforts, working tirelessly on behalf of others. Healthy and always *doing,* she maintains a lifestyle in which volunteering plays a central role. That said, she has received two awards recognizing her time and undying devotion to people and causes. The first was conferred by the University of Santa Monica in 1989 – the "Angel of the Year." More recently, in 2008, she was awarded the "Senior Citizen of the Year" of Santa Barbara County by California State Senator Lois Capps. Her spirit remains indomitable and her life typifies all that is good and decent about human nature. She is an extraordinary woman.

"You care so much you feel you will bleed to death with the pain of it"
-J.K. Rowling

Chapter 8 – James (Age 73)

Cancer is a brutal killer. Relentless and unforgiving, each year this menace, in all its forms, claims the lives of more than half a million Americans. The interview with James revealed a man diagnosed with prostate cancer and he was determined to beat it. Fortunately, his diagnosis came at a time when the toxic cells had yet to regenerate in significant numbers. He has been undergoing treatment for a year and despite a few side effects, his prognosis is for a complete recovery. James and his oncologist are working together to achieve full remission. Arranged by a close friend, I met with James at his home on two occasions. A short, burly man, he was forthcoming about his life story, but his demeanor reflected an understandable caution regarding his future. Although he has reason to be optimistic, the incidence of cancer in his family, including his wife, who died of breast cancer, and his own diagnosis, cause him concern.

The American Cancer Society website states that some types of cancer run in certain families, but most cancers are not clearly linked to the genes we inherit from our parents. Like a loose cannon, cancer strikes at will, inflicting numerous family members in some cases and for some, or no reason, leaves others alone. Cancer cells appear to have a mind of their own. Unpredictable, it rears its ugly head at any time and at any age. Even healthy individuals in the final third of their lives are not

immune. Some people, blessed with an early diagnosis and the best medical care, literally position themselves to fight for their lives to conquer it. Many do not.

James said he had experienced many periods of unhappiness due to cancer-related deaths in his family. His sister and paternal aunt both died of lung cancer, and his mother died at age 47 of ovarian cancer. He was devastated by his wife's diagnosis, but he remained supportive and hopeful throughout treatments which ultimately proved fruitless. His spouse, Evie, was a vivacious, youthful, and optimistic person and James said she was strong, if not accepting, of the inevitable. Her malignancy was terminal and inoperable. "Our children, in their twenties at the time of my wife's diagnosis, were traumatized. Both our families showered her with love, time, attention, and prayers, but to no avail," he stated.

James lives alone save his black Labrador, Max, in a home located on a shady, tree-lined street in Santa Barbara, California. He was alert, mobile, and conversed with clarity. Max followed his every move and lay quietly next to him. He seemed to relax his master, and he appeared to understand what we were talking about. The living room was paneled in dark wood and the carpet was thick, like new. As he motioned me to sit down in a rocking chair, I noticed many pictures on the wall which I would ask about later. James thanked me for my interest in his life story, but questioned why anyone would want to read about it. I leaned forward, smiled, and put my hands up – encouraging him to talk. He began to share details of his upbringing, and I believe reminiscing did him good.

James was born in Buffalo, New York, and was the youngest of four children, his sister the oldest and two brothers. His parents were professionals. His mother was an elementary school teacher and his father a pharmaceutical representative. His family lived in a modest home in a suburban neighborhood, and there was sufficient income to provide all of the basic life necessities.

He doesn't have a clear recollection of his childhood, but does recall he had to share a room with his "squirrely" brother, Danny. "We didn't get along and fought for bathroom time. Danny took long showers and I know he did it so I wouldn't have hot water. Damn him!"

"Another thing, now that I think of it," he stated. "It just wasn't fair that my sister and older brother had their own rooms," he railed. You know the baby of the family often gets the short end of the stick. He was serious about his childhood concerns, but he confessed, "I must admit I was a jerk a lot of the time." We enjoyed a mutual laugh and Max stood on all fours and howled. Too funny!

When questioned about other things he remembered, James quickly replied, "Oh yes, it was frigging cold in Buffalo and in the winter we froze our asses off. We kids lived for Saturdays when we pulled our bedcovers over our heads to keep warm. We were thankful we didn't have to get up and go to school. That didn't last all morning though because even on weekends, our father rounded us up to help shovel snow. I don't miss the weather in New York and feel very fortunate to live in such a mild climate here." I then inquired how he ended up living here. His response provided some interesting details. "Well, my father had a good job in a corporate office in Buffalo, but he was relocated several times. The first moved our family to St. Petersburg, Florida. All of us loved the warm weather there – no more snow, no more shoveling snow, or standing next to the heater. It was great going barefoot, even swimming in the so-called Florida winter. I thought I had died and gone to heaven," he said. He further explained that his mother, Barbara, had no trouble landing a teaching job in town and in the summer while on vacation with the boys, she took them to lots of fun places. James didn't think about it much at the time, but his mother slept a lot and seemed overly tired. Little did the family know that cancer was lurking in the shadows.

James asked if I wanted to walk down the street and have coffee with him at the neighborhood Starbucks. Once we arrived, with dog in tow, I ordered mochas and a cup of water for Max. We sat in comfortable chairs and since we were on a break, I didn't feel it appropriate to ask questions. James wanted to talk. Tearing, he unloaded an emotion he must have been storing for a long time.

"I lost the three most loving and beautiful women in my life to cancer and I still grieve for them." For a few minutes and except for the chatter of people placing their orders at the counter, there was silence. I broke the ice and asked, "Do you want to talk about them?" He nodded and said, "Losing my mother rocked my world. She was my best friend. My father, bless him, eased the pain somewhat by encouraging all of us to talk about her after she died. In family *circles*, as we called them, we shared our thoughts and precious memories. My brother, Thomas, said she treated us all differently, based on our individual personalities. That may not sound like an effective parental strategy, but it worked and we all loved and respected her for it. She knew our strengths, weaknesses, and how we reacted to adversity. My mother accepted and loved us for who we were."

He explained that while traveling in their van on a summer vacation trip, the vehicle broke down in the middle of nowhere in the dead of night. The boys complained and even their father was visibly upset, at a loss for words. Their mother told them to relax and adapt to the emergency. After all, it was an opportunity to learn and grow. "Yes, my mother was a teacher in more ways than one. She always asked, what's the worst thing that can happen when things went wrong? "Her calm, caring nature reassured us all on more than one occasion. I miss her so much," he said.

Driving home, my mind churned like a windmill. Despite a new appreciation of cancer's deadly outreach, I was taken by James' honesty and personal resilience.

Impressed with his willingness to be so forthcoming in sharing tragic circumstances affecting his family, I felt both heartened and sad.

I couldn't help but think of a good friend diagnosed with ovarian cancer eight months ago at age 73, evidence of the seemingly random assault for which cancer is known. In excellent physical condition and of sound mind, with no previous serious illnesses, she was playing tennis when she began to experience severe abdominal pain. Several days later, her diagnosis was confirmed. My friend and her family were shocked. Painful chemotherapy, anti-nausea medication, hospitalization, blood tests and understandable anxiety precipitated a significant reduction in weight, constant fatigue, and loss of her hair. None of these conditions could detour her will, however, and she was determined to extricate the deadly cancer cells in attack mode. Although her cancer went into remission temporarily, taking her and family on an emotional roller-coaster ride, the cancer returned and spread to other organs in her body. Tragically, she recently lost the fight of her life and I still grieve for her. One can't help but wonder why her life was shortened. Her death took a piece of my heart.

Another friend, with whom I worked, died six months ago. A fellow educator and trusted colleague, her death was tragic. However, the story of her lengthy bout with cancer is worth noting. Over a period of nearly 20 years, she fought 3 types of cancer. Those of us who knew and loved her understand fully why her life was prolonged. Courageous, energetic, and always optimistic, she battled day after day, month after month, year after year, with a quiet inner resolve. On the outside, she remained ebullient, almost challenging the toxic cells to mortal combat. As if life-like, the cancer remained present but backed away when confronted with such dynamism and determination. But the final outcome was never really in doubt. The only question was when. Her husband and

daughters waived a funeral and instead invited her adoring friends to celebrate her life at a gathering attended by more than 100 people. Accolades and precious memories were expressed informally and publically, many punctuated with humor. I am grateful that I visited her prior to her death. In hospice care, she could barely speak, but she acknowledged my presence. She was a wonderful gift and leaves an endearing legacy. Sadly, cancer won out yet again.

Some weeks after my initial visit, my new best friend, Max, greeted me at the door, tail wagging, and led me to the rocking chair. He even lay next to me. James smiled and said, "He likes you." This visit I intended to learn more about James' personal biography. But first, I referenced the plethora of pictures on two walls of the living room. Standing, we moved from one to the next and James proudly described photographs of his family – his children, Robert and David, parents on both sides, siblings, nieces and nephews, aunts and uncles, grandparents, and a recent picture of his two adorable grandchildren, Katie, age 6, and John, 4. The picture that touched me was one of James and Evie taken at a local restaurant on the occasion of their 25th wedding anniversary. Sadly, she succumbed five years later and was only 52 years old.

His biography unearthed a man of talent and motivation and revealed the last, and most important, family relocation. The timing couldn't have been better. His sister and older brother had matriculated to Central Florida University upon high school graduation – leaving James and Danny at home. Proudly, James said that in the process he finally got his own room. I couldn't resist asking if he and his brother were getting along at that age. He said things were a bit better although they often pranked each other. James said I wouldn't want to know what they did, but most of their antics involved animals of one kind or another. Both James and Danny were

attending junior high school when their father, John, got the word of his transfer to the corporate office in Santa Barbara, California. James' mother was surprised, but very happy. "What's not to like about living in Santa Barbara," James proclaimed. "The beauty, culture, art, and glorious climate are what the city is all about. I will never leave here."

James and brother, Danny, both attended Santa Barbara High School and after Danny graduated, he traveled to Costa Rica for a brief vacation. He liked it so much there that he stayed and still resides there. "He met a gorgeous woman, married, has five children, and has done well in the import-export business. We don't see each other often, but when he brings his family to Santa Barbara, we have great times," James stated.

In a contemplative manner, James then stated that his future was shaped in a most random manner. "My senior year in high school in 1958 while I was eating lunch, I noticed a Navy recruiter setting up his wares on the quad. I thought, what the heck, and I walked over and picked up a recruiting brochure. The back page introduced me to a naval branch I had never heard of – the United States Navy Seabees. I had always been interested in building things and was actually quite good at it, so I wanted to learn more. I paid a visit to the public library to do some research," he stated.

He laughed and explained that in those days there were no computers, internet, and of course, no google. Somehow, he said, students survived on manual exploration. Grunt work, he called it.

James continued, "I was fascinated by the history of the Seabees and their many contributions in both war and peace time construction in all parts of the world. They went wherever they were needed. There was no draft in 1959 – that would come later during the Vietnam War. I thought it best to pursue higher education and decided to enroll at Cal Poly, San Luis Obispo. I majored in

engineering and the courses, particularly my junior and senior years, made my head spin. Each was technical in nature and a few of my friends, including my dorm mate majoring in liberal arts, told me I was crazy. To become a good engineer, whether in design or building, requires great attention to detail, perseverance, and an acute academic mind. I questioned whether I had all the right stuff. Turns out, I did and a great life was within my reach," he stated.

James then said he met Evie, whom he described as the "a wonder of a woman" at a fraternity mixer and after dating a few months and risking rejection, asked her to marry him. He was surprised when she said yes. "She was an accounting major and had great business and money sense. Since I had neither, she provided a great balance. She was beautiful and intelligent. Her long brown hair and big green eyes were to die for, but I wasn't sure what she saw in me. I felt very lucky. After graduation, we talked about a small wedding, perhaps in Las Vegas. Our parents would have none of it. Fortunately they hit it off and decided on a 50-50 financial split, and of all places, asked us if we were willing to have it at the Biltmore in town. "Willing?" "Yes, were both unemployed and had no savings, but everything worked out perfectly. I know this. Our wedding must have cost a pretty penny, and it was spectacular," he said.

Then, quite unexpectedly, the interview took a U turn. James paused, sighed, looked down simultaneously as Max looked up, and said plainly, "I am much older than my years. I am blessed with precious grandchildren and a pretty good life, but all these years I have carried a burden that has nearly broken my spirit. How would you feel, Mr. Grimes, if you lost the most important people in your life?"

"Terrible," I answered. James continued, "What keeps me going are good memories of our lives before Evie died. My commissioning and training as a 2nd Lieutenant

in the U.S. Navy offered great possibilities." He and Evie went together all over the world wherever James was assigned, and he loved building all kinds of things in the Sea Bees. His wife augmented their income in many different countries by doing income tax returns for both officers and enlisted naval personnel. Both their boys were born overseas and they traveled well. Life was good.

He then said, "I retired in 1992, and have an excellent pension. I stay pretty busy and work part-time in a jewelry store not too far from here. Honestly, you know what keeps me going – besides my little grandbabies?" He stopped and I offered an educated guess. "Max," I said. He then stated, chuckling, "You aren't as dumb as you look." Looking at his canine companion, he went on, "This guy is an exceptional friend. We are growing old together."

Out of respect for privacy and anonymity, I am reluctant to stay in touch with seniors whom I interview. However, at the conclusion of our final conversation, James thanked me for my time and interest in his story and asked me to come back for dinner sometime. How could I not? His invitation was genuine and I believed born out of a friendship that was evolving. As we shook hands at the door, I told him I would contact him. Max, shaking, acted like he was leaving with me but James kept him inside. I waved good bye.

James' life has been filled with both happiness and unbearable grief. Coming face-to-face with the reality of personal loss, he has lived with the threat of cancer which has haunted him day and night for a long time. The battles his wife, mother, sister, and aunt waged and ultimately lost, he fought, also. Now, coping, he has not lost his sense of self. He lives on but the pain remains. Telling his story released feelings bottled up, but our conversations certainly didn't heal him. Softened slightly by the presence of his loyal dog, Max, he was candid, lucid, and informative. I can't put myself in his shoes. No

one can. Perhaps providing him an opportunity to tell his story did him good. Referencing Psalms 1 47:3, "He heals the brokenhearted and binds up the wounds," I submit that his wounds remain. But his resilience, courage, and cherished memories will sustain him for the rest of his life.

"Don't get old. It ruins your health"
-Dorothy M. Grimes

Chapter 9 – Sheila (Age 72)

She was very angry. Estranged by her father for many years and 3,000 miles away, his mental and physical health was rapidly deteriorating. Accordingly, as his only living relative, caring for him was now in her hands.

A friend described Sheila's dilemma to me and subsequently asked if she would be interested in an interview, her story perhaps to be included in this book. Turns out she was, and a day and time was scheduled to meet at the local Coffee Bean. Going in, aware of her animosity, I thought she might project that angst during our conversation, but it didn't happen. On the contrary, she spoke calmly and clearly. In a therapeutic sense, I thought perhaps our dialogue might assuage some of her upset. She assumed, correctly, that I sought background on her life leading up to her father's recent placement in an assisted care facility in Hartford, Connecticut. What she shared was a most penetrating and vitriolic biography.

"I was born in Jackson, Mississippi, and have a vague recollection of my childhood. I do remember my parents arguing about money over dinner. My mom, Genevieve, was a housewife which is not a politically correct term nowadays. My father, Glenn, had an excellent job. He worked for a large insurance company and made great money," she stated. If the breadwinner did so well, why was money an issue? She addressed this next. "My father was a tightwad. Isn't that the case with a lot of people? They make it but don't want to spend it. He

was a chauvinist pig and seemed to delight in put-down statements directed at my mother. I know this hurt her. Very caring and loving, she didn't deserve this treatment. He didn't allow her to work but took issue with her spending what he called *his* money," she explained.

Growing up, Sheila stated that she had a non-relationship with her brother, Ethan. He was an introvert and stayed in his room most of the time, eating all kinds of junk food, reading, and thinking thoughts of who knows what. Her mother tried to ration his food but to no avail.

"I was his exact opposite – loud, outgoing and perhaps a bit obnoxious at times. But my parents enjoyed me and I felt valued. They just didn't know what to make of Ethan. Nobody did, really," she commented." She explained that Ethan died recently and until his death, he had looked after their father which was not a lot of work since Glenn was mobile and mentally alert. Ethan, however, prior to his death, helped move their father into a very nice, affordable venue. I then asked, "What will you do now?" Sheila looked up, frowned, and said she needed a cocktail. We walked a short distance to a bar and grill and as we were seated, she forced a smile and said, "I'm buying. Once I have a few drinks, I will tell you more than you want to know."

As she inhaled a double margarita, she exclaimed, "Damn my brother. He was a young man, 68 but he didn't take care of himself. He was obese, never exercised, and if he could he would have eaten the very couch he spent most of his time on. Listen to me. I am no fashion model and could lose a few pounds – well more than a few, but at least I walk a few times a week. Ethan's weight cost him dearly and I can't say he didn't deserve his fate." Just getting started, I had a tiger by the tail. This was one pissed off woman.

Growing up she recalled moving from Mississippi to a small town outside Hartford, Connecticut, America's life insurance hub. Her dad was transferred to an upper

management position with his company. "I think I was in 4th grade at the time and the cold weather was a huge change from the hot, humid climate we were used to. I sprouted like a weed and was taller and heavier than the boys and girls my age. The boys made fun of me. But an incident changed that. I was a tomboy through and through, which annoyed my male peers. One time a little, skinny kid shoved me at recess trying to impress his friends. I decked him with one shot to the chin. From that point on, no one bothered me again. It cost me a school suspension but it was worth it," she added as she dipped a large tortilla chip into the guacamole dip.

"My dad was very unhappy. He observed that I didn't like to play with dolls or do dress-up; rather, I put on my cowboy hat, spurs, and pointed toy guns at Ethan. Most girls liked to put on make-up and wear their mom's high heels. Not me. He began to distance himself from me, believing I was gay. Duh! Turns out, he was right. My mom loved me unconditionally, but my dad was repulsed with my sexual orientation and to this day, has caused a huge rift between us. But this is his issue, not mine. Like other children of the same persuasion, I didn't understand why I was a homosexual, but I accepted it. Hell, what am I talking about? I am a lesbian. But in my formative years, I didn't advertise it or discuss with anyone so as not to cause embarrassment to my family. And in those days *coming out* was, how do the Germans express it – *verboten*," she exclaimed. The drinks had really kicked in now and she spoke in an increasingly louder voice that turned a few heads at the nearby tables. I milked my glass of Chablis and refused a second though she tried to dissuade me.

I wanted Sheila to eat to compensate for the amount of alcohol she was consuming and suggested we look at a menu. We both ordered fish. I thought she might request another margarita, but she settled for a cup of black coffee. The caffeine caused her hands to shake a

little but her voice slowly returned to a normal tone. At one point, she began to cry and I didn't know how to comfort her. In an attempt to keep the conversation alive, I asked her to describe her education and career.

She was forthcoming and quite detailed about her background – stating that she was an over-achiever in both high school and college, making the most of her organizational skills and conscientious work ethic. She made the Dean's List at the College of William & Mary in Virginia, graduating cum laude in 1966. Sheila was then recruited by corporate head hunters of Pfizer Pharmaceuticals, and was hired as an executive assistant to a middle level manager in their New York, New York World Headquarters. "I thought I was going to assume a leadership role, but my initial disappointment wore off when I learned that the salary and benefits package was substantial. I never looked back," she stated. "I really enjoyed my job. The tasks were challenging and exercised my mind muscles, so to speak. Bosses came and went, but I was the picture of stability and remained in the same position in the New York office for 20 years. Time literally flew by. My professional life was great but my personal life sucked. The personalities of my partners seemed to parallel my own – direct, assertive, and uncompromising. I could really pick them."

Changing gears quickly with the effects of her alcohol consumption apparently diminishing, Sheila railed on Ethan again. "I can't believe he left me in this mess especially since my father liked the dork and the attention he provided. All was working so well." She then leaned forward and asked, "Do I have a right to be upset?" I wasn't sure how to answer and stammered a bit before throwing the question back at her. I asked if she thought her anger was going to alleviate or heighten the impact of her new responsibility. She said she didn't know. But she then posed a question I couldn't duck, wondering if she should call her dad once or twice a week, or fly cross

country periodically. I told her both were reasonable options, but in light of their mutual contempt, I queried how she was going to deal with the negative feelings they had for one another, whether on the phone or in person. She just shook her head.

We decided to end the evening and meet again soon. Although Sheila was understandably upset and frustrated by the situation she found herself in, the resentment and hostility towards her brother and the toxic nature of the relationship with her father were influencing her ability to accept the current circumstance, let alone act on it. Asking me for advice when I had no experience or clinical expertise would force me out of my role as a transcriber. My purpose was to listen, ask questions, and describe events of interest to my readers, and the circumstances of her story certainly paralleled what many caregivers experience. But estrangement from a parent, sibling, other relative, or even a friend has its price. There seem to be more questions than answers in terms of how one copes with it all. Caring for a loved one has its own pitfalls. However, when there has been no contact or personal interaction for many years, in this case with a parent, all bets are off. After all, her father had abandoned her physically and emotionally. It is apparent to me that Sheila has to retool her thinking and adapt to the situation for what it is, not what she would like it to be. Am I the one though to tell her this?

A beautiful, warm day – this time we met in a park near my home. Sheila was subdued and initially wasn't very talkative. I led the way with a question that had been on my mind after the first interview, inquiring about her mother, Genevieve. Sadly, she was killed in an automobile accident and was only 50 years old. Sheila was 25 at the time of this tragedy and she stated that thinking about her brought her both joy and sorrow. "I was away at college and her death nearly invalidated a semester of coursework. I was distraught and inconsolable. My mom

was the only one in my immediate family who really understood and loved me. Fortunately, as I look back, my professors offered solace and gave me the benefit of the doubt with my final grades. I should have earned Ds, or worse but I readily accepted mostly Cs and Bs. I vividly remember watching my father at the funeral and he had a scowl as if my mom had done something wrong. I shouldn't have been surprised. Our relationship soon collapsed and we rarely spoke again," she stated in an almost inaudible tone.

Sheila then said something that surprised me. "I booked a flight to Connecticut and will see my dad. This is the first time in our conversations she referred to him in a personal, respectful manner. We spoke briefly on the phone yesterday and he said he was glad I was going to visit. These words of welcome struck me funny. Was he losing his mind and had forgotten about shutting me out of his life? If so, then I guess he is no longer accountable for his behavior," she said abruptly. She then indicated she had a conversation with the resident physician who told her that Glenn was mobile, alert most of the time, but had recurring lapses in memory. Accordingly, he had been recently placed in the memory loss unit, requiring 24-7 nursing care.

I asked if she wanted to make things right with him and she stated that wasn't going to happen. "I have been told that time heals all things, but I have been rejected and hurt deeply by this man. He remains a monster – with or without dementia. If he knows of what he speaks, then he is playing with me, but I am not certain he realized it was me on the phone," she stated. Referencing the physician's comment, Sheila was probably right.

This situation is an interesting, if not disheartening, dilemma. If Glenn is in a state of progressive dementia and is losing his ability to recall events, time, and people, then what and how can Sheila communicate with him? Can she in good conscience give

him a clean slate, letting him off the hook for his horrific behavior? As his new caregiver, can she justify accepting him as is and ignore their history of bad blood? My conclusion, in the simplest of terms, is that it is what it is. Sheila will do what she believes best knowing that the hate she carries will not be acknowledged nor the relationship with her father reconciled.

The two conversations with Sheila spent us both emotionally and physically. The story and the circumstances of her life, particularly regarding her mother, brother, and father weigh on her heavily. Not unlike what many other individuals have experienced with a parent or other relative, there are more questions than answers. Caregiving, even under pleasant conditions, is challenging enough, and despite rejection and abandonment by her father, she will find ways to cope and move forward. Her patience, resiliency and willingness to forgive her father will be put to the test. Time will tell.

"Caregiving is rewarding but not enjoyable"
-Anonymous

Chapter 10 - Reflections on Caregiving

My mind conflicted with contrasting emotions. On one hand, I felt great admiration for the kind and loving care the wife was providing her husband. But I was now suddenly struck by an ominous realization. A hospice volunteer, this was not the first time, nor would it be the last, that I would experience such feelings. My patient's physical condition was deteriorating and here I was leaving a home where his family was worn by anxiety and coping as best they could with the prospect of his inevitable death. On the other hand, I was ready to enjoy the rest of my day. Some worry about where their next meal is coming from. More important, however, will my friend be blessed with the gift of another day?

A cliché, albeit a soft one, often verbalized in conversations reacting to a death or a grave circumstance, "Each day is a blessing," rings true. Death now, in my eyes, is very real. When speaking with my patient today and looking deep into his eyes, I couldn't help but think this man could be me.

For many baby boomers with aging parents, caregiving becomes a way of life; a full time pursuit, if you will. Lacking training or preparation for such an important endeavor, they learn as they go. But even if one is up to the challenge, the road is fraught with unexpected twists and turns. Researching and writing this book has heightened my understanding and appreciation of a world

I couldn't have possibly imagined just six months ago. Seeing first hand a loved one or friend slipping into an abyss is very painful. There is no joy in it. Those of you who are (or have) been a primary or a secondary caregiver understand that, despite good intentions, the time, energy, and expense, to care for another is both demanding and exhausting. That said, caregivers who work find ways to provide what is needed for their loved one. An excerpt from the *American Association of Retired Persons Bulletin* (November, 2013) titled, "Your Family," offers strategies utilized by caregivers to maintain ongoing employment, either full or part time, while tending to a family member.

A woman interviewed for the article stated, "Working caregivers like me are everywhere. Some of us are open at work about our caregiving roles, but others keep it to themselves. Those who don't disclose their caregiving situations may do so for personal reasons, but many keep quiet because they are concerned about repercussions at work. Working caregivers are in the position of keeping (or finding) work while meeting the constantly changing needs of the people we care for. We never know when a crisis is around the corner." Sound familiar? Some ideas shared that will help juggle the balancing act include: telling your employer, changing work hours, telecommuting ("remote work" from the loved ones' home or another office), and taking leave. Utilizing any or all of these suggestions require energy, flexibility, and, in the end, an empathetic, supportive boss."

For many seniors, place of residence is a transitional pathway. Solitary or partner-shared living may require some or minimal care. As physical and/or mental capacity diminish, placement in a long-term facility such as assisted living, a group or retirement home, extended nursing care, a veterans' venue, or a memory loss unit become necessary. Depending on a

variety of factors including, but not limited to, mobility and individual preference, "home" is not an option. But "home," the connotation of which means different things to different people, becomes a powerful and conflicting word. As dementia limits the ability to recall, think coherently, and perform what once were simple tasks, "home" is no longer relevant. I spoke with several seniors residing in a long-term facility who, openly and, at times defiantly, expressed their desire to leave although doing so is unrealistic in terms of the care they require. On one occasion, while visiting a friend's aunt in an extended nursing facility at lunch time, I overheard a man seated at a nearby table say, "I need to figure out how the hell to get out of here." His tablemates chuckled, but he wasn't joking. Residing in a location often not of their choosing, his statement evidences the confinement seniors' experience.

A starting point is this. When does one need care? The answer varies. A man residing in my mother's assisted living facility, only 55 years old – young by today's standards, has congenital heart disease and bone deterioration that severely hamper his mobility. No relatives are available to help him. He will remain in a facility for the rest of his days. Not a happy picture. Interestingly, several staff providing care for him are age-wise his senior. In stark contrast is a woman I observed at a local Costco. Standing in front of me in the pharmacy pick-up line she appeared to be in her late 70s or early 80s. I heard the clerk ask her date of birth. Responding quickly, she stated, "10-10-20." I was astonished. This woman was 94. She wrote a check, spoke clearly, and walked away from the counter with ease and energy. Could she have driven herself to the store? Is she actually caring for someone, perhaps her own child, spouse, or other relative?

Another example of the spirit driving longevity was featured in a local television human interest segment. A woman was celebrating her 105th birthday with family and friends in an assisted living facility and offered advice on aging. "Eat your vegetables, keep your nose out of other people's business, and enjoy each day as best you can," she lectured emphatically. Laughter then rocked the room. Her words exemplify the power of positive thinking and the drive to do all things necessary to maintain a healthy, prolonged life. In a different way, she was offering care and love for those responsible for her welfare – a reversal of roles. She played it well.

Caring for a loved one at their residence can be particularly challenging. In addition to the normal housekeeping chores such as cooking, cleaning, and paying bills, more serious matters need attention on a regular basis include making doctor's appointments – transport to and from offices, conversing with physicians, and regulating medications. Reminders, either verbal or in written form, to the special person regarding when and how the prescribed drugs are to be ingested is an important undertaking. I learned much about how this works as a result of a chance encounter with a female baby boomer.

Taking my patient to a clinic for physical therapy is a hospice task and while sitting in the waiting room on one occasion, I struck up a conversation about this book with a nice woman named Katherine. She was completing an intake form for her mother, seated across from me. Aging, as you might expect, was the topic. Her mother, 101 years old, was having pain in her ankle, necessitating a physical therapy regimen. Katherine asked what the book was about, and I told her the text consisted largely of interviews with seniors. She stated, "You should interview my mother. She has led a very interesting life." I took her up on the offer and we exchanged phone numbers. A few

weeks later, the three of us met at Katherine's home, a two-story residence in uptown Santa Barbara.

In the living room with Katherine seated at the computer table and her mom resting comfortably on a large, chesterfield chair, I began asking questions – hoping that the information she provided might be of sufficient interest to include in the book. Anyone living 100-plus years surely would have a family history, stories, and events to capture the willing attention of readers. But she was either unable or unwilling to communicate any amount of detail to my questions and appeared uncomfortable in my presence. Katherine repeated my inquiries so the questions were clear – but to no avail. Directing my statement to both women, I said, "Perhaps we can talk another day." Katherine's mom, appearing confused, stood up and walked downstairs to her living quarters.

At this point, Katherine sat next to me and apologized for her mom's non-responses. I told her I didn't want to be the source of her mom's upset. Katherine and I talked for a while and then she led me to the front door. I asked her if her siblings (three brothers and a sister), all of whom lived out of state, called their mom and if they were supportive. Her answer shifted my thinking in terms of interviewing her, rather than mom, to add depth, meaning, and personal experience to this chapter. She said, "They call but never ask how I am doing." This comment remained on my mind for some time. As I walked down the brick stairs to my car, I couldn't help but think – who cares for and supports Katherine?

We arranged to meet over dinner in a few weeks. Weeks turned into several months, but the conversation we would eventually have over dinner on a warm, summer night revealed a truly compassionate, giving, and loving daughter. Among other things, Katherine talked about the difficulty she had been experiencing in monitoring her

mom's decreased mobility and mental acuity. She described the event that necessitated her mom's placement in a nursing care facility. In the middle of one night, Katherine, asleep in the upstairs bedroom, heard her mom yell for help downstairs. She had fallen in the bathroom and suffered multiple bruises to her legs and thighs. Thankfully, however, no bones were broken. Katherine immediately called 9-1-1 and the ambulance motored both women to a nearby hospital. Caring for her mom in-house had become unmanageable. Unable to continue caregiving under the present circumstances, she stated that her mom is now quite happy in a facility and the pressure is off them both. The change is doing both good.

Supervising and tending to the needs of a loved one with dementia is extremely challenging and frustrating as symptoms of mental deterioration are difficult to read. Researching, consulting with physicians, nurses, or friends in a similar situation are helpful. But the cues we receive from loved ones are difficult to interpret and the language they use is often contradictory and illogical. While visiting my friend Emma's aunt in a memory loss unit, I came face to face with a dark side of the mind. In her private room the conversation consisted of Emma's verbal responses to statements or questions posed by her aunt. Family and intimately acquainted with each other for years, a question came out of the blue. Her aunt stated, "I don't think we have been properly introduced – who are you?" In this instance, how does one respond? I have learned through observation, hospice training, and personal experience that verbalizing an answer to a question of this nature would solicit recall, which is neither productive nor appropriate. Oftentimes, a non-response is best or, better yet, redirecting the conversation with questions or statements unrelated to the initial inquiry. Either way, trying to correct or clarify her aunt's question would serve no purpose. We have to meet individuals struggling with recall where they are, not where we wish them to be –

preserving their dignity rather than trying to be right or prove a point.

I was seated now and a few minutes later a woman, a resident of the unit, suddenly entered the room, looked at me and said, "You are adorable. I love you." We three collectively smiled – acknowledging the levity in the woman's words. Her behavior, although sad and quite random, broke the ice. If we allow it, humor can serve as the best medicine, regardless of where or when it occurs. There is no logical way to understand the inexplicable behavior of loved ones suffering from memory loss, but treating them in all ways and at all times with kindness and respect is paramount.

My hospice training emphasized the importance of conversing in the present with no references to past events. During one of my first visits with a patient, I made a rookie mistake. We were talking about food, admittedly one of my favorite subjects, and I asked what the gentleman had for dinner the night before. He responded, "Hell if I know." Oops! Lesson learned.

Finally, most caregivers possess a wonderful sense of self and characteristically display fortitude, resiliency, adaptability, and compassion. That is who they are. For all those individuals who serve in this capacity, we are most grateful. They are gifts to humanity.

Final Thoughts

Apocryphal or factual, storytelling is often magical, creating images, past and present which ignite food-for-thought. Stories are both ageless and timeless. Those shared by seniors interviewed proved to be very compelling. Some were very fascinating. Often mesmerized by detailed descriptions of people, places, and things, I frequently put my pen down and just took it all in. Turns out, I discovered that listening attentively to what was being said was exhilarating. Most expressed their gratitude that someone cared enough to listen. After all, how often does someone give us their undivided attention?

Everyone has a story but the opportunity to tell it is frosting on the cake. Take the kindergarten student eating mac and cheese at dinner who unexpectedly blurts out, "Hey mom and dad. I told my teacher today she had a pretty smile." Mom then commented, "That was a nice thing to say. Good boy." End of story – short but sweet. But seniors, possessing a lifetime of events and experiences, store voluminous amounts of information waiting to be unlocked and shared. In *Old – Stories of Aging and Reflections on Caregiving*, it was an honor to examine inside and out many interesting, surprising, uplifting, and heartbreaking tales. Like turning the pages of a great book in eager anticipation of the words yet unread, I excitedly gave my full attention to the vignettes shared.

Although I sought to obtain views on aging, death, and dying, asking each senior to describe their life experiences without restriction to specific questions created a free-flowing and spontaneous dialogue. As one might expect, health issues, family struggles, personal highlights and lowlights, dominated the conversations.

The vicissitudes of life, the apparent random nature of events, and the impact, positive or negative, of individual choices made by each helped gain insights into their personal character and added a depth of meaning to what was shared. Many undervalued the importance of their accomplishments when it was clear they had impacted events and people more than they realized. But they left little doubt they cherished the relationship described, particularly family. That said, recounting their stories became a self-actualizing experience.

The final chapter recognizes and celebrates those individuals who give their time, talents, and energies in caring for another. Motivated by not only a sense of duty, but also a desire to make daily living both comfortable and meaningful for their loved ones, the tasks they perform, willingly and unselfishly, elevate the dignity and worth of all for whom they care. They are heroes.

Initially, I planned to include a postscript at the conclusion of each chapter. Typical of my training and professional background, I believed writing a summation would be helpful to the reader. For weeks, I struggled with the teacher in me as I wanted to address the question, "What did we learn?" Several friends advised me against it. I resisted at first. One friend told me to trust readers to draw their own conclusions. Accordingly, I acquiesced. I let the stories, not my opinions, speak for themselves. The treasure chest of information uncovered was priceless, the content of which challenged us all to think how we can make better our own lives.

Bibliography

American Cancer Society website, *Genetics and Cancer*, 2014

Bell, Virginia & David Troxel, *The Best Friends Approach to Alzheimer's Care*, Health Professionals Press, Inc., Baltimore Maryland, 1997

Graham, Billy, *Life, Faith, and Finishing Well*, Thomas Nelson Publishers Inc., Nashville, Tennessee, 2011

Lama, Dalai, *Advice on Dying: And Living a Better Life*, Atria Books, New York, New York, 2002

Payutto, P.A., "Aging and Dying," Talk delivered on 4/22/96 to an International Symposium on Death and Dying (https://budda.net)

Scott-Maxwell, Florida, *The Measure of my Days*, The Penguin Group Publishers, New York, New York, 1968

Zelinski, Ernie J., "The Retirement Quotes Café – Aging and Old Age." (https://retirement-quotes)

"Old Age by the Numbers," New York Times (https://oldage.blogs), 2010

"What Does the Bible Teach us About Angels?" (https://christiananswers.net), 2009

"Allison V-1710," (https://wikipedia.org), 2011

Alzheimer's Fact Sheet, National Institute on Aging (http://alzheimer's Publication), 2009

American Association of Retired Persons Bulletin, "Your Family," November, November, 2013

"What Me, Marry?" Widows Say No, New York Times (https//:nytimes.com), 1992

***Webster's New Collegiate Dictionary*, G & C Merriam Company, Springfield, Massachusetts, 1981**

Ecclesiastes 1 ESV – "All is Vanity" – Bible Gateway (https://biblegateway.com), 2010

https://thinkesist.com.quotations/elderly

"New Clues to a Long life," National Geographic, May, 2013

442nd Infantry Regiment, (https://wikipedia.org), 2011

Japanese-American Interment, htttps://wikipedia.org), 2010

Slaves and the American Civil War, (https://wikipedia.org), 2010

https://Geneaology.Archives.com., 2013

https://openbible.info/topics/getting into heaven

"Reinventing in the Third Age – Older Adults and Higher Education," American Council on Education, Met Life Foundation, 2012

https://seniorsourcecolorado.com/Boomers Leading Change, 2010

CDC – Cancer – Statistics by Cancer Type, (https://cdc.gov/cancer.htm), 2009

About the Author

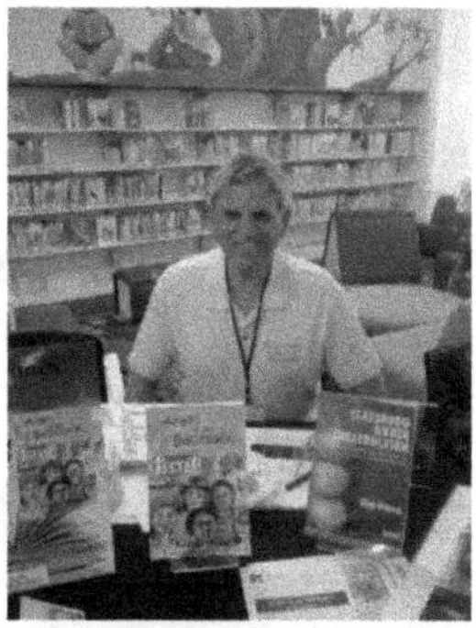

Rich Grimes is an author, poet, university professor, and proud father of two adult daughters and grandfather to three adorable grandchildren. A retired high school principal, he remains active in education – teaching, conducting staff development workshops, writing articles for professional journals, and posting educational topics on his blog. Recently, he served as an Administrator on Special Assignment at Redondo Union High School in Redondo Beach, California.

***OLD – Stories of Aging and Reflections on Caregiving* is Rich's third book. *Classroom Under Construction* (published in 2006) continues to be a very useful instructional tool for both beginning and veteran teachers and *Angel in my Backpack* (published in 2013) is a fictionalized series of short stories about schoolchildren and the human angels who touched their lives. He authored a poem, *Flight 93* in 2003 commemorating American heroes of 9-11, for which he was awarded "Distinguished Recognition" by the International Society of American poets. Venturing into a new genre, he is currently working on *Animal Friends*, a children's book based on his poem of the same name due for publication later this year.**

Rich earned a B.A. degree in History from Chapman University, and an M.A. in Educational Administration from California State University, Northridge. He is a hospice volunteer for Visiting Nurse and Hospice Care in Santa Barbara, California, devotes much of his time mentoring aspiring and first-year teachers, and enjoys playing tennis. Rich resides in Ventura, California.

www.ingramcontent.com/pod-product-compliance
Lightning Source LLC
Chambersburg PA
CBHW052044270326
41931CB00012B/2620
* 9 7 8 0 9 9 0 5 8 8 6 0 3 *

PAREJA, TRAUMA Y EDIPO

La dificultad de las parejas para vincularse

PAREJA, TRAUMA Y EDIPO

La dificultad de las parejas para vincularse

VICTORIA ELENA CASTAÑÓN DE ANTÚNEZ

Primera edición 2015

©ARCHITECTHUM PLUS S.C.
Díaz de León 122-2
Aguascalientes, Aguascalientes
México CP 20000
libros@architecthum.edu.mx

ISBN 978-607-9137-38-0

CONTENIDO

NOTA DE LA AUTORA:

Los ejemplos clínicos citados en este libro son una recopilación de conflictos de pareja vistos a través de muchos años de práctica clínica y no se refieren a ninguna pareja en específico. El objetivo de ejemplificar conlleva exclusivamente fines didácticos y es responsabilidad de la autora que escribe este libro.